Blogging for Happiness

Blogging for Happiness

A guide to improving
positive mental health (and wealth)
from your blog

Ellen Arnison

NELL JAMES PUBLISHERS

Copyright © 2011 by Ellen Arnison

All rights reserved. No part of this book may be reproduced or transmitted in any form or by any means without written permission of the Publisher.

Published by Nell James Publishers
www.nelljames.co.uk
info@nelljames.co.uk

British Library Cataloguing-in-Publication Data
A catalogue record for this book is available from the British Library.

ISBN 978-0-9567024-3-2

First published 2011.

The Publisher has no responsibility for the persistence or accuracy of URLs for external or any third-party internet websites referred to in this book, and does not guarantee that any content on such websites is, or will remain, accurate or appropriate.

Note: The advice and information included in this book is published in good faith. However, the Publisher and author assume no responsibility or liability for any loss, injury or expense incurred as a result of relying on the information stated. Please check with the relevant persons and authorities regarding any legal and medical issues.

Printed in Great Britain.

For CNA
because he never left a day unseized.

Contents

Introduction 1
   What is a blog? 4
   Why blog? 7

How a blog can create happiness and improve mental health 17
   Thinking positively 17
   Letting off steam 25
   The blogging community 28
   Achievement and creativity 40
   Knowledge gained 43
   Doing good for others 48
   How blogging can help in the real world 52

How to blog 59
   Where do I start? 59
   What should I write? 62
   How do I get followers? 69
   Technical tips and design ideas 72
   Statistics and rankings 77
   Competitions and awards 80
   Remaining anonymous 85
   Legal issues (copyright, libel) 92
   Blogging dos and don'ts 93
   Using Twitter 103
   Making time to blog 110

Blogging for money 113
   Advertising 114
   Advertorials 116
   Affiliates and working with brands 118
   Reviews 120

    Business blogging   122
    Online 'expert' CV   125

Resources   127
    Got a question?   127
    Bloggers recommend / quoted   136
    Bibliography   138
    Useful websites   138

Index   141

Introduction

I knew I was in trouble when I was handed my newborn baby and, while I pretended to be interested in him, all I wanted was for someone to take him away. Then I couldn't shift the idea that there was something seriously wrong with him and no one wanted to tell me.

Before then, mental illness was something that happened to other people. Clearly, I was strong and tough and a coper. Of course I was. It was simply a matter of gritting my teeth and getting on with it, like always. Anything else was just a manifestation of weakness, or so I thought. It wasn't that I was unsympathetic to people with a mental illness, I didn't see how it could happen to me – if I didn't let it.

I supported a close friend through a difficult bout of depression. But then she'd always had it, at least through the 20 years I'd known her, and things would be better if she'd just take the pills. However, it did make made me realise that mental illness could infect an intelligent and rational brain and turn it, temporarily, into something totally different.

Fast forward to my third pregnancy. The first two were some years previously and reasonably unremarkable. Subsequently I'd left my sons' dad, struck out on my own, found someone else and, dear reader, I married him. So far, so happy ever after.

Then my dad died, quite suddenly in his mid 60s from lung cancer. We had fewer than ten days from his diagnosis to his death – nowhere near enough time to get used to the idea, say goodbye and get accustomed to the reality that people you love do actually die no matter what you want.

In the right order of things, we all come to see the end of our parents' lives sooner or later. But it doesn't matter how commonplace this loss is, the grief and adjustment is still painful. More so, perhaps, when it comes as the first whiff of real hard 'gosh-it'll-happen-to-me' mortality.

And so it was for me. In the spirit of never knowing what's around the corner and not wishing to leave regrets, my husband and I thought that, perhaps, it might not be sensible, but another child would be lovely.

At my age – the menopausal side of 40 – I knew there were tricky statistics that said it was riskier, less lucky. So I held my breath until 12 weeks' gestation and took all the tests. Ha. Everything was fine and healthy – stick that into your increased risk due to age calculator. I knew it would be OK. And so I relaxed, even began to enjoy it. Told the kids, our friends and the wider world. A few more weeks went past, apparently, I was blooming.

Until one day there was a spot of blood. Hardly anything, certainly nothing alarming. Enough to ignore, 'probably nothing at all, but come and have a scan anyway'.

But the scan told another story. The baby was dead and had been for a couple of days. Perfect, just dead. So then there was the unpleasant matter of delivering her through a dark, memorable night in the company of ghosts.

The loss of an unborn baby is the strangest, most raw thing. You say farewell to the baby that's growing in your imagination as well as the one in your womb. And as if jousting with the grief and adjustment isn't enough, you've got to untell people your happy news. Meanwhile, your body hasn't caught up – hormones rage and you can't get back into your non-pregnant clothes. It's enough to shift even the most stable person off their axis for a while.

The post-mortem examination revealed that I had a blood clotting disorder that caused the tragedy. When pregnant, my blood was too sluggish to flow properly.

Still, always one to make the best of it and hearing something ticking not so far away, I was undeterred. Luckily, I was pregnant again within three months – not bad for someone of my advanced years. But it was tense.

In truth it was a miserable pregnancy. I had to inject myself with blood thinning drugs hoping they – and will power –

Introduction

would keep my blood flowing freely. Every day some new discomfort would emerge as if my body was paying penance for the healthy growing life. And it was healthy and growing, so I couldn't complain, could I? No, especially as I knew many people were not as lucky as me. They lost babies and didn't get another chance. They just had to come to terms with it.

And so the day came and my third son – big and lusty – was delivered. But I didn't want to know him. I suppose if the fog had lifted long enough, I would have rationalised that getting to the point of giving birth to a healthy baby had taken all my reserves of everything: my job was done. However, there was nothing rational about those few weeks in June 2009.

I've done this before, I told myself, I know how to look after a new baby. But then I just couldn't work out what was wrong. I didn't know how to stop this colicky baby from crying, I couldn't get him to put on the required amount of weight and I certainly wasn't able to give my other two children the attention they needed. In short, my family was turning into a bit of a nightmare.

'Get on with it, it's just the baby blues,' I scolded myself, through tears. 'You wanted this baby so much, you can't complain now.'

Then less than two months after the baby was born and before I'd had time to regain anything like my normal composure, the ground beneath my feet shifted again. My brother died suddenly, at the age of 38 while out on a run. He left a widow and two pre-school sons.

It's hard to describe the next few months without resorting to cliché – going through the motions, vale of tears, on autopilot, struggling to stay afloat. I was so wrapped up with my misery I worried that my children would be affected. How could I give them what they needed when I could barely get through a day?

It was a relief to be diagnosed with depression. Suddenly, it wasn't my fault I couldn't cope and I certainly didn't have to recover all by myself.

The antidepressants and the counselling helped, but something else helped my recovery. Something that I had abandoned a while back with my normal sunny self, yet became one of the most effective tools to my recovery. My blog.

What is a blog?

A blog can be whatever you want it to be, there really aren't any rules. It's easy to assume that in this switched-on, plugged-in, wi-fi world that everyone knows what you're talking about when you say you're a blogger. However, it wasn't that long ago that confessing to having a blog would just cause, at best, shrugs and bewilderment and, at worst, have people edging away and looking for an excuse to leave.

So what exactly IS a blog? It is an online diary or journal. But the content doesn't need to be literary – it can be videos (vlogs), images or audio.

Hands up anyone who kept a diary as a teenager, especially one with a tiny key that you kept on a chain or under your pillow? Yup, me too. And I've kept diaries at various other spells too although over the years when life got really interesting there were fewer and fewer entries. This has certainly changed with a blog. When a lot is going on, I can't wait for a chance to sit down and have a good blog about it.

In the main this is a function of maturity and that 'interesting' doesn't automatically come along with late nights and hangovers (although I wouldn't rule it out). The change has also come because I now understand – and crave – the function that writing a blog post has for me. It helps the mental digestion by consolidating my thoughts. It also helps hugely to have my nebulous notions pinned down under the gaze of other people.

In one respect you could say a blog is just another place to put 'Dear Diary, today I had pizza for tea and met P on the way to school. He's lush. I love him'. But that's only one of the many facets.

A blog is updated chronologically with the most recent posting at the top. And that's it really.

Introduction

As I said, it's your blog, you can make it out of anything digital that you fancy. Blogs often feature an element of interactivity such as places were readers can comment. And there's usually some method of keeping up with new posts – a way of signing up for news of fresh material.

The biggest difference to a diary is that, to some degree it is public. Other people are going to read it and not when you are old and everyone who you've written about has shuffled off. They don't have to find the tiny key under your pillow and sneak in for a look. By publishing a blog you are inviting them over and leaving it wide open at the most recent juiciest entry.

So, in a nutshell, this is a blog. A public online diary or journal where you can share your thoughts, insights and news and invite others to comment and discuss. Still interested in how this can help your mental health? Good!

It might help at this stage to consider where blogs came from. While similar on many levels to journals, diaries, newspaper columns and photo albums, the combination is still relatively new. So while running the risk of giving an egg-sucking lesson, I'd ask you to indulge me in a look back to the 1990s when the first web log was so called.

Apparently a hairy American chap called Jorn Barger began logging the internet in 1997. Barger wrote essays and discussed Artificial Intelligence, James Joyce and Kate Bush, although perhaps not all at the same time. He used the internet to record the things he came across. His idea was to create a mesh – or web – of resources created by linking to other pages or sites. Barger's 'web log' notion was being picked up by others and copied, and by the beginning of 1999 there were 23 in existence. Can you imagine it? By early 2011 there are 156 million and I believe several dozen more at least are created every hour.

In early 1999, Peter Merholz, founder of Adaptive Path, a consultancy specialising in internet user experience, joined the gang and decided he was going to call his 'we blog', which was quickly shortened to blog. A verb was hatched. And the rest, as they say, is history.

Although it wasn't really. Merholz and Barger were all about sharing the things they found rather than producing their own material. Back then, community outweighed blog content. Some early bloggers tried to maintain a list of all the other blogs and their posts, but the whole field was expanding so rapidly it quickly became impossible. Rebecca Blood, author of the *Weblog Handbook*, said: 'Weblogs are no panacea for the crippling effects of a media-saturated culture, but I believe they are one antidote.' An antidote to the crippling effects of a media-saturated culture? Rebecca wrote that in 2000.

Only this year in 2011, Lord Richard Allan, Facebook's director of policy for the EU, echoed her when talking about Facebook's slightly Orwellian ambitions to create a layer across the web where someone's Facebook profile and information go with them to whichever corner of the internet they feel like visiting. If the notion of a government-sponsored national identity card scheme where all our information hunkered down on a tiny little computer chip was a little unsettling, then what of the idea of a commercially-sponsored scheme where all our information hunkers down on a tiny little bit of Facebook? World domination plans aside, Allan clearly knows his web and how it works. He said: 'There are two kinds of internet. The information web is where people search for specific facts. Then there is the social web which has no purpose. There people spend time looking at things, sharing pictures. People come across information and discover things. Blogger was the first experience of a social web.'

Blogger.com was created – in the opportunistic way of the web – to capitalise on a trend by providing a free blogging vehicle so you didn't need to be in the least bit technical to blog. And now there are many ways of doing the blog boogie, almost none of which require any special knowledge.

Introduction

Why blog?

In many ways it's not possible to separate 'what's a blog?' from 'why blog?' – the two go together like a desperate writer and a well-worn simile. For me 'why?' is perhaps one of the easiest bits to deal with. Because I can.

I've always been a scribbler of one form or another. As a kid I used to write diaries, dog-eared volumes of revelations along the lines of 'watched TV, did my homework, had tuna for tea'. Student days were more like 'Sorry Diary, I was too drunk to write last night', clearly no Samuel Pepys then! More personal revelations might include 'walked back from class with x, I really fancy him'.

But all along I had the notion that One Day someone would find my diaries and publish them in a great hoorah of publicity. In fact, I know there is a box somewhere in my house full of those jottings. You'd have thought that if that was the ultimate fantasy I'd have tried somewhat harder on the readability front, wouldn't you?

So for me, blogging was a simple extension of keeping a diary and being able to fast forward the bit where other people get to read it. However, what started as a simple literary (very small 'l') knuckle cracking exercise quickly grew to have many facets.

It became somewhere to share memories and photos with friends and family members, it became a vehicle for starting a discussion and it taught me many things, introduced me to some fantastic people, earned me money, got me a couple of pieces of work and helped me through one of the blackest patches in my life. Not bad for what began as a minor indulgence.

Rebecca Blood, arguably one of the first bloggers and likely the first woman, began her blog *Rebecca's Pocket* in 1999. She said: 'The blogger, by virtue of simply writing down whatever is on his mind, will be confronted with his own thoughts and opinions. Blogging every day, he will become a more confident writer. A community of 100 or 20 or three people may spring up around the public record of his thoughts.

'Being met with friendly voices, he may gain more confidence in his view of the world; he may begin to experiment with longer forms of writing, to play with haiku, or to begin a creative project – one that he would have dismissed as being inconsequential or doubted he could complete only a few months before.'

Thank you Ms Blood, I'll get my coat...

But she's right, in the same way talking about an issue can clarify one's thoughts, blogging about it crystallises opinion beautifully.

Consultant clinical psychotherapist Terri Bodell specialises in life skills and she explained how it works: 'It's largely the benefit of writing it down. The medium isn't important. Whether you're writing it in a blog or a diary it makes really no difference, the fact is you're writing it down – you're getting it out.

'I'd say when you're writing it down in a diary no one is actually reading it but that's not necessarily a better thing, sometimes it isn't. Sometimes it's good to have the feedback of others in a blog.'

This makes sense. For example, I hadn't really considered my thoughts about being a feminist. Or at least, the ideals had become so bent out of shape by child rearing and giving up exhausted on the notion of 'having it all', I hadn't thought of it for years. Then I was invited by blogger Ryan Wenstrup-Moore, also known as *Transatlantic Blonde*, to take part in her regular Feminist Friday parade. She asked when I first knew I was a feminist.

Here's what I wrote: 'Well, it makes me furious that men get paid more than women for doing the same job. I rage that women become insignificant at work once their work-life juggles become conspicuous. I think it's just crap that some girls aspire to be only someone's wife. (I'm not saying that being a good wife/mother/homemaker isn't important and sometimes difficult, but it's hardly splitting the atom. In my book, kids should start off with the loftiest goals and work down.) It also makes me cross that some men really, really, deep down don't think women are their equals – it's almost impossible to prove (and why should we) but you just know.'

And I recalled how a first reading of the *Women's Room* by Marilyn French brought all the messy thoughts about men, women and parents to one place. Now I look forward to Ryan's calls to arms.

You see, it actually feels as if I'm able to make a difference, albeit a minute one. When I was free and available enough to be an activist – I didn't bother fighting for women's rights. I wasn't hindered by children and, then, I had neither tried to juggle everything nor been far enough up a career ladder to see the ceiling.

But when I finally got it – like a great many women – I was too sleep-starved and busy just keeping it all going to have anything left to try to change things. Now though, I can stand up – or rather sit down at my desk – and say I'm a feminist and, even better, I find it's only one of the many benefits to blog keeping.

Blog benefits have come from all quarters, many of them not something I could have imagined when I first signed up to Blogger and rolled my sleeves up. After the first few tentative steps, and the months where my blog simply meant my mother and my siblings didn't need to phone because they already knew what I'd been doing, I began to realise there were people out there. And that was the first big change for me. Other people were reading what I'd written. You'd have thought that this wouldn't be a new sensation to someone who has been in journalism one way or another for far too many years. But it was.

You see, in newspapers, even when you know the circulation is however many hundred thousand, sitting in the office, it's hard to maintain the idea that even a few of the hundreds of thousands are going to read what you created. It's easier to persuade yourself that they might only buy the paper for the sport, the crossword, the telly listings or the bingo.

And in any case, the only time you're sure someone has read your piece is when they phone up to complain, usually at length, about it. When was the last time you thought 'that was an interesting, well-written and carefully researched article, I must call to congratulate the journalist'?'

So to have someone comment kindly on something I'd written was such a buzz. Once I figured out how to read the statistics that proved that real people actually came to my blog and stayed there for a while, I was delighted. OK, it was a tiny fraction of the numbers that might read a newspaper, but these ones were mine. Hardly a stellar achievement but I had got a handful of people I didn't know to spend a few moments of their busy days clicking around my blog. It's hard to explain how thrilling that is at first. It's a similar sensation to the first time you sit on public transport while the person next to you reads an article you wrote. The temptation to lean over and say 'that's me' is almost uncontrollable. I suspect my writings are a bit like an aspiring singer or dancer who can't keep themselves off a stage. It's like the least obvious form of showing off, but showing off it undoubtedly is.

However, an ego tippytap on a keyboard is far from the only reason to take to blogging. The next big blogpiphany – it's my book, I can invent words if I want – came when I found the Britmums group. It's one of the first times I had found a proper community that I knew I could be part of. Not that I wanted to spend my time discussing the colour and consistency of poo, nor would I really call myself a mummy blogger, but I loved the way the women – and men – of this group wrote and shared their lives.

Here was somewhere I didn't have to explain myself and the reasons why I might choose to share the minutiae of my existence with, potentially, the whole world. I imagine it's a bit like the moment when you find the sport you're going to be good enough to get to the Olympics with, or write the tune that the *X-Factor* winner's going to sing or invent the next gizmo that's going to have the Dragon's cheering in their Den. Not of course that there's a blogging Olympics as such, but I knew I could hold my own. And it wasn't about being able to construct a lyrical sentence or use long words; it was because I fitted in with what was already being said.

So, blogging helps people locate and tune-up their voice. And for me that was unexpected. When you write for money, in the main, you write on the topic and in the style you're being paid for. You aren't the authority, merely the vessel through which information is passed. It's a rare privilege to get paid to suit yourself in print. So the sensation of being able to write what the heck I liked was extraordinarily liberating.

For the first time in decades I felt I was being properly creative. For many of us creativity is something we left at the school gates. Beyond decorating the odd cake or deciding what to plant where, it's not easy to let the products of your imagination take flight.

Confidence and achievement coach Dale Rockell said: 'Creativity is stifled too much. Kids want to be creative adults but then we're stuck in this go-to-work, do-that way of life and creativity is just not allowed to flourish. Blogging helps people with their creativity.'

It certainly does – the sheer breadth of talent and imagination on the pages of blogs never ceases to surprise me. There are stunning photographs, proper snort-your-coffee funny posts and thoughts and observations that can take your breath away.

My blog as a place to air my thoughts was especially important when I began freelancing and, while I could still say what I liked, there was, generally, no one at home to listen to it. So, in part, my blog was merely an exercise in water cooler chat.

I suspect my husband was delighted with the arrival of my blog. Previously when I was working at home, he'd arrive back from his day's labours exhausted and in need of some peace and quiet. I, on the other hand, would be equally tired, but desperate for a chat with a grown up. Until he learned to look like he was listening sympathetically, it caused a bit of tension. So my blog afforded me the sensation of being surrounded by adults whenever I wanted them. And posts on a subject my dear husband would have to pretend to care about needed trouble him no longer.

And liberation is a driving force for many bloggers. Often it's a place to say what they can't elsewhere in the real world. Many isolated people – whether by accident or design – find blogging gives them contact that seems to go much deeper than than necessarily superficial world of Facebook and Twitter.

I wonder if some bloggers get drawn to it because it's the thing to do at the moment. Their friends have one and they feel left out. Sandy Calico, who blogs at *Baby Baby*, said: 'I started my blog because everyone else seemed to have one. Now I blog because I've rediscovered a love for writing. I also blog because I love the blogging community. Mummy (and daddy) bloggers are such friendly, accepting, interesting and helpful people. They make me laugh, cry and nod in agreement.'

Bloggers are also created from separation. From gap year kids to explorers of the uncharted, through the magic of the internet, families and friends can keep in touch with their adventurers. To a great extent a blog leaves blue airmail letters and post restante addresses redundant. Just blog it – use video and photos if you like – and mum knows what you've been doing. Or at least your edited highlights.

Equally expats' blogs allow the folks back home to know what everyday life is on their foreign shore.

Blogs are born to chart pregnancies, babies, to catalogue recipes, to record crafts created, to test out creative writings, to share mountains climbed, theories tests and religions explored.

Some blogs pop up when someone finds themselves in a niche, particularly one they didn't ask for. There are a great many blogs about medical conditions, for example, and they form strong support networks.

Others again come to the sport looking for support or a friendly ear when they are going through a turbulent time.

Alice Castle is the *Dulwich Divorcee* and her blog has now spawned a successful book. She said: 'I started my blog in 2006 just after splitting up with my husband and coming back to live in the UK. I'd been in Brussels for eight years before that. I didn't know many people in my new area and blogging was initially just a way to vent my frustrations as I went through a very painful and difficult divorce.

'To my surprise, though, I found I was getting comments at the end of blog posts from people who were sympathetic and understanding. I was astonished as I really hadn't thought for a second that people would be reading my ramblings. I found it very moving and encouraging. Some had been through similar difficult times themselves, some were just kind enough to empathise. It helped me keep going through the process and my blog soon became a source of solace and support.

'Over the years the emphasis of my blog has changed as I have moved on from the divorce, but I will never forget what a great comfort it was to discover there were people out there whom I had never met, but who still cared about me and my travails.'

Other blogs are created as part of a marketing plan. They drive traffic (website visitors) and spread the word about a business. If that's the only motivation, they'll possibly fizzle out soon enough, but many bloggers got a taste this way and were as hooked as the rest of us.

Author of *Realmshift* and *Magesign*, Alan Baxter began his blog, *The Word*, as a means of promoting his published fiction, but soon it became an end in itself, especially for a solitary writer, an antidote to an insular way of life. He said: 'My novels and short fiction are competing with so many others out there these days that authors need to have an online presence to get themselves noticed. There's an assumption that authors will be available to some extent, sharing their process and interacting with their fans. I've grown to really enjoy that aspect of writing, which is otherwise a very insular occupation.

'I've also grown to really appreciate blogging as an outlet beyond my fiction writing. My blogging usually focuses on the writing, publishing, storytelling aspects of life – my own and others – and I greatly enjoy the interaction with people, both professionals in the field and fans, that blogging encourages.'

Kathryn Brown who blogs under the pseudonym *Crystal Jigsaw* writes about her life as the wife of a farmer, the mother of a child with autism and a newly published author. Hers is a strong voice in her online communities and she spends a lot of time encouraging new bloggers by reading and commenting on their sites. She said: 'I had one of those conversations recently with someone who doesn't understand blogging. When they said it was something they'd never be interested in, I asked why. Their answer gave me ammunition, even though I would never judge anyone's reason for having an opinion.

'Fake friendships was mentioned, together with "couldn't be bothered reading about people who I'll never meet". I tried to explain that at least 95 per cent of the bloggers whose blogs I read, I know I'll never meet them, but it doesn't mean I find their lives less interesting. She didn't want to listen and shook her head, whilst I tried my best to think of something to say to convince her otherwise.

'So I showed her my blog. I let her read some of my posts and look at the photographs I've published over the last four years. She couldn't believe it, had no idea how incredible having a social life online can be. I felt really proud afterwards, telling her about the many blogs I have the pleasure to read and all the amazing people I've come into contact with.

'She never realised how much effort it takes to keep a blog updated, and interesting enough to pull in the readers, the most exciting part, I told her. Whether or not she'll start her own blog I don't know, but it reminded me of when I was first introduced to blogging and couldn't believe how rewarding it could be. But the best thing was, after half an hour of telling this person how much enjoyment I get from blogging, I've made someone realise that having a social life online is something to be embraced, not laughed at.'

Kathryn is passionate about blogging, but blogging is often borne out of a passion. A hobby or enthusiasm can readily spill out onto the keyboard in a blog post. Some bloggers relish another outlet for their favourite topic while others want to transmit their message in the hope of setting things straight and shifting others' beliefs.

Political activist and fan of popular TV, Caron Lindsay has a blog called *Caron's Musings*. 'I didn't, however, want it just to be dry, political analysis as some political blogs were. I wanted it to have a lighter feel, reflecting all my interests from *Doctor Who* to *Strictly Come Dancing* to Formula 1, with a bit about family life and parenting thrown in too,' she said.

'It's also been a good discipline in encouraging me to find out more about policy, go back to the roots of where my political values come from and put them down in ordinary language.

'I also wanted to show, particularly in the wake of the expenses scandal, that people who are involved in politics are human beings like everyone else and that in the vast majority of cases, are decent people whatever their party.'

Caron's urge to show the world that political people are human too is interesting. It hits the nail on the head for many bloggers who are inspired by a desire to lift the lid on something in their lives and show the human face of it. And it's that human face that is at the heart of a good blog.

I have a bit of a notion to categories blogs into different types: hobby blogs, family blogs, political blogs and so on, but actually doing so would do blogging a disservice. There are thousands of reasons why people blog, but ultimately we do things because we like them and they give us something back that we want. Blogs will do that for you by the bucket load.

How a blog can create happiness and improve mental health

Thinking positively
'Happiness doesn't depend on any external conditions; it is governed by our mental attitude.' Dale Carnegie

From early on, American author and poet Maya Angelou was a heroine of mine. In the first part of her autobiography, *I Know Why The Caged Bird Sings* she tells of living through rape and racism but refusing to become a victim. She took the most awful experiences, wrote beautifully about them and, most importantly, learned from them and used them to fuel her work. The first time I read one of her books, it crystallised how I felt. 'That's me, I won't dodge bad stuff, I'll use it to learn from' and I became a bit of a Pollyanna. Just like the heroine of the 1913 children's novel by Eleanor H. Porter and subsequent Disney film starring Hayley Mills, things usually turn out fine and I can find the best in everything. The 'real' Pollyanna plays what she calls The Glad Game where she must find something to be glad about in every situation. At times, for me this has even appeared in the extreme version, which may be known in some circles as self delusion.

That's how I knew during the months after my third son was born and my brother died I was more than just a little low. That time was the most painful and foggiest I've ever crawled through. Pollyanna had fled, leaving in place a tense, shrivelled creature for whom the sun never shone.

I was really worried about my children, for a while I hated them too and that just wasn't fair. While I don't think less-than-perfect motherhood is to blame for every child's problem, I do believe that mum has to function reasonably well.

So I started forcing myself to find one single solitary positive thing to record about each of them every day. And slowly, slowly it worked. I found myself seeing what they did and thinking 'lovely, that'll make a funny/charming blog post'. I spent more time with them looking for things to record. Gradually I fell back in love with them and Pollyanna returned.

And I'm not alone in believing about the power of positivity and blogging. Former magazine editor Keith Kendrick, who blogs at *Chronicles of a Reluctant Housedad*, found his blog helped him to cope after he was slung into the position of being a stay-at-home father due to redundancy while his wife went back out to work.

The move was very hard for him and required a shift in attitude that seemed impossible at first: 'The nights were dark and my entire outlook for the future was based on gloom; when every thought I had was about me; when every emotion was a maelstrom of self-pity, self-indulgence, self-flagellation and, well, selfishness,' he admitted.

'I looked inward, not out; failed to see what I had; was incapable of imagining the potential for fulfilment there could be. I obsessed with my purpose in life as being an ability to provide, not to parent. I felt weak, pathetic, pointless, useless and – to my eternal shame – resentful.'

Things began to change for Keith with the launch of his blog. He committed to the internet every painful step from the bitterness of waving his wife off to her exciting new job to dealing with the tedious, tedious daily routine. *Chronicles of a Reluctant Housedad* allowed him to air his misery somewhere safe without necessarily dropping it corrosively at the smart shoes of his wife when she returned home from her day of work.

'And instead of feeling isolated and trapped in my new role, I felt supported, encouraged and connected. I've never met any of the people who contact me, and perhaps I never will, but these new "virtual" friendships mean a hell of a lot to me,' he added.

'It is, in part, because of them – because of their comments on my blog posts, their engagement with my tweets – that I now feel very happy to reveal the five words I thought I would never, ever say. I love being a housedad.'

So Keith's blog started off as somewhere for him to have a right good whinge, yet turned into a source of affirmation and joy. Another blog success story. I must say that writing about something you really love – however that might be clouded in the short-term – can serve to underline the positive and reinforce the strength of feeling. And if you can find something funny, charming or cute to say then that's even better.

Happiness coach Thea Jolly, who blogs at *Talent For Living*, said: 'Smiling is one way to reduce the distress caused by an upsetting situation. Psychologists call this the facial feedback hypothesis. Even forcing a smile when we don't feel like it is enough to lift our mood slightly.'

So the message is to write your smiles down, even if it takes a huge effort to haul your virtual cheeks up your digital face. I know life can't always be a bowl of cherries, bed of roses or whatever metaphor you prefer, but our existence is rarely so bleak that there isn't the smell of fresh toast, a ray of sunshine, a cheerful greeting or a happy memory to sit with for a while. Even experts in grief acknowledge that it's impossible to bear the weight of the awfulness of loss every minute of the day without a break. That's why, often, there are hysterical giggles from the bereaved – it's nature's way of saying: 'Put the load down, just for a moment.' Equally in the bleakness of deathbed gatherings, there can be glimpses of joy. The days by my dad's bed as his life was ending were precious and filled with love.

Don't worry, I'm not going to insist you join me down here on the yoga mat with your legs crossed. I'm just pointing out that if you look hard enough there will be something – however small and fleeting – that's a source of pleasure or satisfaction. Sometimes it can be incredibly difficult to spot that tiny flash of positive and that's where a blog comes in.

Consultant clinical psychotherapist Terri Bodell said: 'People who are depressed, whether post natal depression or any form of psychological down-ness I'd say tend to only perceive bad. Things always look black or bleak – they never see any upside. When I talk to someone in my practice who's depressed or going through depression I'll say "has anything good happened this week?" And they will invariably reply "no, nothing". Then I carry on talking to them and all of a sudden I'll find that a neighbour popped in with a casserole for them or the person in the supermarket smiled at them.

'It might be small, but does it really mean nothing went right that week? It's very easy to get into that mindset when you're feeling down about anything. You don't need to be clinically depressed just having a down day and it feels as if nothing is going right.'

Bad luck comes in threes, they say. And have you noticed how it seems to and how when something goes awry, suddenly, everything else in life is a source of misery and gloom? Conversations become a litany of dreariness? So, then, perhaps unsurprisingly people don't leap to join you when they know all they're going to hear at lunchtime or in the pub is your whingeathon. So then you're Norma-no-mates for whom everything goes wrong.

And with no one to talk to and a whole load of disasters under your belt, you start to tense and brace yourself for the next thing. Will things be off when you open the fridge? Will your car fail to start in the morning? Does that diversion mean you'll be late? And that cloud mean it'll pour? The meeting with your boss means you'll be sacked, become destitute, lose the house and eventually starve.

OK, you've seen where I'm going with this. Expect rubbish things to happen and they will because you're looking for them. Conversely, be sure fortune will smile and you'll be pleased when it does.

I know this sounds simplistic and naive, but it even has a fancy name. Terri explained: 'This is called the Law of Expectation. Have you ever had the situation of thinking about buying a car and you'd plumped on a car you'd like to buy. Within the next week you'll see about 50 because your mind is on that kind of car

'Glass-is-half-full people always look for the positives. Does it mean that everything always goes positively in their lives? No. But if you start looking for the positive, it makes you more upbeat. If you started forcing yourself to look for a positive, your mind would automatically start looking for more of them.'

Terri's recommendation for a more positive outlook is to find at least one upbeat thing about yourself and your life every day. Obviously the best thing to do with that thing, from my point of view, would be to blog it. In fact, while Terri thought I'd done quite well with writing positive things about my kids, she said I should really have been dishing up a daily goody about myself too: 'I would have liked it if you'd give one positive about yourself too. I would have immediately said put one positive thing or one thing you are personally grateful for.'

Terri explained it's about balance, something of a mantra for the psychotherapist. She prescribes a long (but not too long) hard look both inside and outside in search of, you guessed it, balance: 'It's the same process whether it's internally or externally. You can't do one without the other. If you're too internally focused you'll be much too naval gazing and I know coming from a psychotherapist that might sound a bit weird, but I'm a little bit more pragmatic than many. You can't naval gaze because it doesn't work, but equally, you can't look outside yourself for everything. People who do that are never happy.'

So how do you find this balance or virtual smile then, when the world is conspiring against you and you've just got a parking ticket?

I'd say, first of all, is it funny? If you can write about your disastrous day or catastrophic camping experience with humour that makes others – and ultimately yourself – laugh then you're half way to putting it in perspective.

After all, it's hard to imagine anyone is going to enjoy reading your catalogue of everyday unhappiness unless you've added something else to it. If I don't know you I'm not sure I'm going to care too much about your broken washing machine, stubbed toe, chicken poxy child, bitchy boss or tenacious spare tyre unless you tell me about it with humour.

I'm not saying don't have a moan, by all means, be my guest. You'll certainly feel better for it, but just don't expect crowds of readers rushing back for the next installment of your mundane miseries.

How about something you've gained or learned from the ordeal? Was there an upside? Did the traffic jam on the way home mean you saw a sensational sunset? Did your broken tooth mean you avoided the toffees and now you've lost half a pound? With the exception of what I call proper negative events – bereavement, divorce, serious illness, etc – the silver lining is often fairly easy to spot.

Maybe all you got was a valuable lesson. It could be you learned something that means the exact same disaster will not befall you a second time. I take delight in writing blog posts around a slightly tongue-in-cheek list of things I've learned from whatever the topic was. The next time something hideous or horrible is happening, try it.

Terri would perhaps advocate a 'things I'm grateful for today' or 'ways in which I'm blessed' approach. Blogging through adversity does help maintain perspective, or balance, as Terri would have it. Caron Lindsay, who blogs at *Caron's Musings* and continued to do so even during a lengthy bout of ill health, said: 'Blogging, and maybe taking a day or several days to write a post, helped keep me focused and occupied. It meant that a physical illness did not become a long term bout of depression as well.

'There were days I could write nothing – and could only manage a few tweets if that. There were better days when I could do a bit more – but whatever, I was able to keep in touch with a world outside my four walls. That made life a lot better for me.'

Another blogger, GP Sheonad Macfarlane credits her blog, *Touch and Tickle*, with great things. Among other things, it deals with how Sheonad and her family cope with her toddler daughter's diagnosis of spinal muscular atrophy, which is a genetic disorder that affects nerve cells so that muscles can't be used and become atrophied.

Sheonad said: 'Blogging has, honestly and sincerely, saved my life this past year. I find myself in my blog. In the peace and quiet I can withdraw and have room to explore and reflect. I don't have to hide there; my feelings are open and raw and real.

'I can find inspiration between the words of my blog and I can follow my journey from heartbreak to present day. But most importantly, for me anyway, I can share my journey with others so that they don't feel so alone during their times of need: they can see that there is a future full of hope and joy and happiness to be enjoyed.

'As a doctor I will often recommend keeping a diary as a way of mapping a patient's mood or diet or even when they are trying to conceive. By recommending diarying the person will start to pay attention to themselves, to their day and, hopefully, in time find the answers that they are looking for; answer that we are looking for so that we can move forward to helping them.

'Today, in the modern world with technology abundant, blogging is coming to the fore as another way to take stock of ourselves: to map our moods and tell our stories, to journey towards happiness and contentment, to find support from others and share our story. I cannot recommend it enough.'

Are you a worrier? There are times the usual concerns start to become somewhat wilful. The perfectly understandable mild ponderings about the future – how to pay the bills, how to stay healthy and what's around the corner – can get a little stroppy. They start popping into your head when you don't want them there and generally being bothersome. Even when you know they don't actually bite, the bark can be alarming.

Having a good old blog about worries can work wonders – it gives them a slap and sends them back where they belong. Mental health charity Mind advocates list writing as a way to tackle worries. They suggest the following: 'Try writing a list of what's troubling you. Use statements, rather than questions. Instead of, "What will happen if I don't get there on time?" say,

"I am worried that I won't get there on time". This focuses on precisely what the fear is.'

Susanne, who blogs as *Ghostwritermummy*, started her blog as a response to the difficult nature of her son's arrival. A traumatic labour ended with Susanne under a general anaesthetic and her baby delivered limp and blue. Consequently she found it difficult to bond with him and she suffered insomnia, anxiety attacks and flashbacks to the delivery: 'My GP seemed unable to help me and the waiting list for counselling was so long that my son would be at school before anyone was ready to listen to me.

'I sought support from wherever I could and ended up writing for my local NCT newsletter. One of the ladies there suggested I started a blog. At first, I didn't want anyone to read it but, slowly, I began to rebuild a little confidence and I began to involve myself in the community.

'When I published my birth story, I was overwhelmed at how many other women contacted me to tell me their story. I published a birth trauma page and invited some fabulous bloggers to share their stories with me. I began to open up about what had happened to me. People close to me began to read my blog and to understand a little about things that had been happening since my son was born.'

This chimes loudly with me. If you have a healthy baby in your arms, it's almost impossible to find someone to listen when you need to talk about the way he or she arrived. My eldest boy was born in the Canary Islands by emergency caesarean section. For a long time I couldn't clear my mind of images of being rushed down a corridor to an operating theatre, the noise of the instruments being used in my belly and having my arms tied down to hold me still. Back then in 1999, I'd never even heard of a blog but I knew I had to write my experiences down. And once I had done it I felt like a weight was lifted. The memories of those traumatic hours are still with me, but I've been able to put them into their normal place instead of allowing them free reign in my mind.

Susanne and another blogger, Jayne of *Mum's The Word*, started a new blog called *Maternity Matters* which is about and for people who have suffered birth trauma. Susanne has come up with a list of tips for would-be bloggers who are considering a little online therapy.

- Write it. Get it down on screen and you may find that's enough. I have many posts sitting as drafts that have closed a chapter for me and don't need to be published. Yet.
- Get involved in the community. Get your name out there and accept the support that will come your way. There are so many other bloggers out there who have been through what you have and if they haven't, they will be willing to read about it and offer support anyway.
- Write for yourself. Don't worry about making your readers depressed or want to turn off. Your blog is your own and you don't need to apologise for what you write.
- Don't be afraid to ask for help or to get involved in other organisations. Contacting the Birth Trauma Association and setting up *Maternity Matters* has been one of the most beneficial things I have done. One voice is rarely loud enough – a whole host of bloggers just might make a difference.'

Letting off steam
This section could also be called the blog as safety valve. There's so much steam being vented onto Wordpress and Blogger and their ilk that if someone was really clever they could harness it to solve the fuel crisis. So how useful is a blog as somewhere for a bitch, moan or rant? If you subscribe to the idea that anger must be released and resentment allowed to drain away, then yes, in spades.

How many times have you heard: 'I need a rant'? It's hugely satisfying to let fly about something that has rubbed you up the wrong way. I've had a blast over incompetent service, attitudes that irritate and people who really get on my wick. And it does feel good – it's off my chest and onto the screen with a huge sigh of relief.

Being mostly a jolly sort of person, I tend to try to disregard minor irritations as if they were small flies. Although my sweet-natured husband would probably suggest that on occasion I can be a 'right stroppy cow', I really don't understand where he gets that idea. I endeavour not to let them trouble me and, in turn, I don't tend to trouble them. But, sometimes, after swatting the fly away a few dozen times, I find I've got a bit cross and this irritation just spills out.

Lately, it was the number of people who seemed ignorant to the fact that certain newspapers publish provocative articles online for the very function of provoking people into reading, reacting and sharing their anger. I had a good rant about how ignorance meant the outraged who, with each tweet were, in fact, helping the paper they profess to hate.

Several times, I've been unable to control the urge to blog my infuriation at women who make sexist comments about their useless men. Oh, and I've had a few goes in staunch defence of tabloid newspapers. It could just as easily be shoddy service from a big company, blatant attempts to cheat or someone in the public eye who isn't playing straight. That said, most of the time my blog is a virtual vale of sun-dappled grassland... really. It's just foul-smelling blobs of rant are likely to appear from time to time. And they really are rather fun to write.

But many bloggers are so certain of this ranting function that their blogs don't seem to do much else. *Dr Rant* is written by a group of seemingly embittered medical staff who want to have a say about the NHS and beyond. It's an excellent example of professional frustration finding an outlet. Whether or not it is read by those in high places is almost irrelevant as it almost certainly makes the author feel better.

Dr Rant warns: 'Some readers may find the use of foul language offensive, for this we apologise in advance. *Dr Rant* thinks people dying in the NHS because of political interference and lack of funds is offensive. You decide which is worse.' Angry stuff. He's among friends too. There is a wide raft of medical bloggery, most of it furious and all of it anonymous. Other professions – teachers, lawyers and local authority staff have spawned a similar stack of cross and venting blogs.

Sometimes things in the newspaper industry have got up my nose so much that no amount of tutting or sighing loudly will get my point across with any kind of satisfaction. Then I've had to blog – poor reporting, declining standards of grammar, the use of idle clichés or, even, broadsheet writers who think themselves above the rest of us. It takes grumbling about conditions and personalities at work a level up from having a bitch in the staff kitchen or by the water cooler. It may, even, do some good.

Whistleblowing is really only a step up from rantyblogging and in both cases the motivation is frequently white-hot fury. It's just that whistleblowers are persuaded they are spilling the beans from the moral high ground for some greater good.

Do you remember the anonymous insider who claimed that all was not as it seemed behind the glitz and music of the latest raft of reality TV talent competitions? The writer was so incensed by the alleged manipulations and machinations of the management intent on producing good telly at the same time as groom performers to be milked like the proverbial herd of cash cows in the future. The showbiz mole was determined to dispel the idea that the hugely popular series had even the slightest thing to do with finding the best talent. The post was picked up by the press and caused a minor ripple but may have opened a few people's eyes only a little wider than before.

And as far as the frustrations of daily life are concerned, the humble blog has done a lot to reduce cruelty – in the form of kicking – to cats. So someone swiped your parking space, next door's dog left a great steaming 'present' in your garden or, my current rant fodder, a mobile phone provider that seems to think a four-figure bill for data roaming for three days abroad is reasonable. The festering bubble of impotent rage that sits somewhere between your collar bone and your breakfast will turn to corrosive bile if it doesn't find a way out. So blog.

PR consultant Mike Ritchie blogs at *There Comes A Time*. When numerous things get his dander up – whatever his dander is – he puts it back down again with a good blow out on his blog: 'I think a blog offering can be a useful, inoffensive and controlled way to let off steam – and not just for the hell of it, either. The letters' pages in national newspapers, in particular, have been outlets for outpourings from the committed, and those who should be committed, for a very long time.

'When I rant about something – usually bad manners, lack of respect and courtesy, gobbledygook English, bad spelling/grammar, and booking fees – I don't expect any solution at the end of it, I really don't. The best I hope for is that any reader can find something to agree with, or even take exception to. Along the way, I hope they enjoy the read, too.'

Interesting that Mike is keen to make sure that his rant is seen as a short-term blast at something irritating rather than a huge issue with which he is struggling. Blogger Jax Blunt from *Making It Up* has thought about setting up another blog in order to give herself a safe place to let it all hang out: 'I've considered setting up an anonymous blog for ranting. Having to explain yourself and smooth ruffled feathers kind of takes away the stress relief of getting the rant out of your system in the first place.'

Ultimately it is good for the soul to let off steam, but there should be caution too. See the sections in chapter 3 on legal issues (pages 92–3) and blogging dos and don'ts (pages 93–103).

The blogging community
'With blogging you can have the support of a coffee morning, whenever you need it.' Suzanna Scott

I'm not a team player. I don't think of myself as a community person, I'm not joiny-in and I don't often volunteer for stuff. In the street we live I'm on smiling and nodding acquaintance with everyone, but rarely have a longer or deeper conversation than the routine one about dog poo. It's the way I like it (the conversations that is, not the dog poo).

But I'm probably unusual in that. Most people, apparently, want to be part of a bigger something, want to feel at home and familiar. Many years ago, I had a boyfriend who claimed the *Cheers* theme tune *Where Everybody Knows Your Name* was his favourite all-time song because of the sentiment. It tinkles along about finding a place where people are pleased to see you and everyone there knows you and your story.

If *Cheers* is before your time, I'll explain. It was an American sit-com set in a Boston pub where a group of dysfunctional locals meet to bemoan their lives. The charm of it was that in the bar, the locals all knew and accepted everyone's funny little ways but didn't like them any the less for it. One of the characters, Frasier Crane spun off to a hugely successful series.

It's an appealing idea – whenever you wander into 'your' special place, there's a friendly face, someone who knows your story and a sense of belonging. Over the years in various transient communities in different parts of the world, I've had places that felt like that. However, since the arrival of children and an arguably more grown-up lifestyle that has, on the whole, gone.

I expect there are people who can still go to their local pub and be sure someone will ask them 'what's up?' and care about the answer. But for a great many of us, for various reasons, just don't do that any longer. We have babies requiring sat, we're new in town, we're too skint to afford a drink, we're working through AA's 12 steps, we are too shy to make the first move or we simply don't know where to start. Sometimes, even if we do muster the courage, we can't get a word in edgeways.

The modern world can be a lonely and isolating place. It's a cheerful coincidence that my blog was born in the same week I started my life as a work-at-home freelancer. While I tend to be quite happy, possibly happiest, by myself all day, my husband was the first to notice I needed some other people in my life. He would come through the door after a hard day in a busy newspaper office and I would be lurking nearby waiting to share witty conversation with him. All he wanted to do was sit in silence with his mouth slightly open.

At first my blogging voice was fairly weedy and I was doing little more than writing for my three pals and my family. At that point my husband didn't read it, snorting down his nose in a derisory way when I mentioned it. For quite a long time, I don't think I even knew anyone else was blogging. Of course, I knew bloggers existed and I did read other people's blogs but I didn't feel I 'knew' anyone out there.

Then I found the BritMums community (although in the spirit of the dear old BBC I must point out that 'other blogging communities are available'). This is a place where parent bloggers in the UK come together online. At first I was astonished by this group of parents who wrote these articulate posts, many of which resonated with me and who also seemed to know each other. Then I noticed a 'come on in' kind of message and saw a few other newbies taking their first shaky steps.

So with a deep breath, I dived in. I had found one of the online blogging communities where it feels everyone is 'glad I came'. The more I blogged and the wider the scope of the subjects I wrote about, the more other communities I came across. There are, of course, as many communities as there are subject that captures people's attention.

In Canada there is blogscanada.ca and topblogs.co, in New Zealand there is kiwiology.co.nz and Australians can start at blogs.com.au. Then there is the mighty BlogHer.com, community in America that has 24 million visitors a month and lists 22,000 blogs.

I get involved in the ScottishRoundup. A weekly blog edited by a team of volunteers that attempts to collate the best of what's being blogged in or about Scotland. Through it I 'know' writers whose subjects are as diverse as politics, the outdoors and places to go for a drink. I'm also in the parents of autistic kids community, the freelance journalists community, the people who climb hills community and probably several others.

How a blog can create happiness

BritMums founder Susanna Scott had spent quite a lot of time 'talking' to bloggers from her native America. She blogs at *A Modern Mother*: 'I started the community in 2008 as a place where parent bloggers could virtually meet, gather and share ideas and support each other. When I first started blogging, there were loads of US-based bloggers, which was great, but bloggers are social people and I was looking for local bloggers to get to know in person too.

'A few of us met at a Chuggington [UK kids' TV show] launch event and we were commenting on each other's blogs, but we really needed a place where we could have conversations .... That is when BritMums was born. It's grown to more than 3,000 UK-based bloggers.'

As a spin-off, she, along with Jennifer Howze, who blogs at *Jenography* and formerly was The Times' *Alpha Mummy* and Sian To of *Mummy-Tips*, organised the Cybermummy conference, and high-profile parent blogger events seem certain to feature in the UK every year. Press coverage of the event pronounced on the 'rise and rise of the mummy blogger'.

Membership of BritMums is increasing and the number of newly hatched parent blogs seems unlikely to drop soon. However, Susanna is keen to encourage the BritMums community, both on and off line. 'Nothing will ever take the place of a physical community,' she said. 'However, online communities can be great support networks, especially if there is a component that includes real life meet ups (this really helps online relationships, as it is easier to be respectful to someone if you have actually met them, and there is less of the bitchiness, hide-behind-the-laptop stuff).'

Tracy T blogs at *Beadspaperglue*. She found BritMums helped her develop her blogging muscles and the strength of her voice: 'Yes, I would say I have definitely, in my short time here, felt the community, whether on Blogger, Twitter etc, everyone has been lovely and supportive. I am so glad that I found the BritMums' site as a "base" so to speak.'

There are as many blogging communities as there are communities in the real world and, similarly, they are just as diverse: geographical communities, groups of sports supporters, political activists, animal lovers, people of faith and music lovers to name a tiny few.

There's huge value in simply being in the same space – virtual or otherwise – as like-minded people or those who are going through the same experiences. This is obviously going to be of greater benefit if the community, by definition, consists of isolated individuals. You won't, therefore, be surprised to find thriving groups of home educators, people who work at home and those who end up many miles from their original communities such as ex-pats and military families.

Isolation is rife. Consultant clinical psychotherapist Terri Bodell said: 'In rural areas there are a lot of small villages and you can get stuck – particularly with kids. Because you don't have transport or money you can be stuck, you can also get stranded because of depression or ill health. Even the weather can mean it's hard to get out.

'And then who do you talk to? Blogging can be a life-line for the lonely. People don't talk to their neighbours any more, it's not like it was 20 years ago. My mother used to have friends round and they'd have a cup of tea and chat. That's where they used to divulge, disclose, offload and talk. Now we're all too busy and separate.'

So blogging communities can also serve the same function as a having a neighbour who will drop in for a natter and to dispense some sympathy. Like neighbourhoods of the information superhighway. That's lovely then – but is that all there is to it? A glorified tea party?

I don't think so. These online communities provide much more than an exchange of ideas or an internet measuring tape for your life. As with any community, it's about support. In the case of blogging it can range from the equivalent to a subtle nod of recognition to a huge great sloppy kiss of love and some hand holding.

I'm not sure that this is the place for a discussion on the collective power of human will and how, in my opinion, when people meet (however this happens) with purpose, there is often far more going on than the sum of the individual contributions. There are no doubt specialised blogs out there for that. However, few would dispute the fact that there are frequent cases where strength of will defeats the expectations of science.

Confidence and achievement coach Dale Rockell said: 'For example, if someone is dealing with something gravely serious like cancer and is blogging about their experiences, it's there for people to share and empathise with. And when you create that sort of support, people start feeling better.'

This, according to Dale, is a variation on the fairly common phenomena that when someone is diagnosed with a life-limiting condition, family and friends tend to arrive offering their support. And then these patients sometimes outlive their prognoses because of all the positive energy coming their way.

'They feel better because everyone's around them,' Dale added. 'They're not thinking of their illness. This happened to a friend of mine. They said she only had a couple of months to live but she went on for a year because the whole family was around the house every day and doing things they weren't before.

'So it's the same with a blog, it's a feeling of having shared experiences and feelings ... particularly when bloggers and readers start having conversations about it.'

Obviously, I'm neither suggesting a blog can cure the likes of cancer nor that the benefits should be confined to those hellish times when dreadful illnesses are diagnosed. But I will venture that the life-enhancing benefit of a community bring a little extra oomph to any blogger, whatever their circumstances.

Terri said: 'Connecting with others certainly does help people to deal with emotions they're feeling and to bring them into a more positive mindset. It's an effect you can't beat.'

So everyone agrees that we are social animals who need each other – one way or another. But a small note of caution must be sounded that an online community must not replace all forms of interaction in someone's life.

Eva Cyhlarova, head of research at the Mental Health Foundation, said: 'One of the fundamentals of good mental health is social interaction. To an extent the internet encourages meaningful friendships and social connections, and this can be a positive influence on people's lives. However, our *Lonely Society?* report indicates that communicating via the internet doesn't provide the face-to-face contact that really benefits wellbeing. Therefore, while technology can help us to keep in touch, it is no replacement for face-to-face human interaction.'

My eldest son has Asperger's Syndrome and so I'm drawn to the blogs of other parents in a similar situation. I believe human nature is always keen to find someone going the same direction, either for company or to race against. One of the well-known behaviours of people on the autistic spectrum is to become obsessed by things. My dear boy has had his fair share – starting with the jigsaws and then the train toys. However, these days the subject that is filling his head, tends to be the one that is also filling our ears. I was finding it particularly difficult. On the one hand I firmly believe that being listened to is hugely important for kids yet taking in what my son was saying was becoming impossible. I was either fobbing him off or pretending to pay attention. I realised what I was doing and it was starting to make me feel unhappy. If I treated any other child like that it would be downright mean. Should I simply try harder, or what? In the end, I blogged about it. For me, writing things down has always helped to clarify the thought and work out exactly what the problem is and, it would do no harm, to see what anyone else felt. Within minutes I had several bloggers – from the supportive autistic parents' community – giving me feedback. Oh yes, they understood, I wasn't doing anything wrong. And they filled my comments box with support and suggestions. The community of parents with kids with autism is reasonable clear-cut, as are the communities of the parent bloggers, politicos or the football enthusiasts of whatever persuasion. However, the story here isn't just about finding an established community you fancy and knocking on the door. You can start your own community. Clearly following in Susanna's footsteps and becoming the leader and a host of a big group such as BritMums requires time, energy and confidence. But it's not the only way. As in real life, groups of blogging friends and acquaintances come together for other reasons. Some spring up around a shared experience, from a meeting, or simply because the members enjoy it.

If you're not sure where your community is, ask yourself if you routinely visit the same blogs, do you look out for their posts, perhaps you make a comment and, maybe, the blogger replies. They are your community. That's the crux of blogging: it's a two-way thing. Say hello, make a comment and before you know it you've got a community going on.

Community can evolve from conversation and relationships. Writing a post that responds or is inspired by something someone else put on their blog is a start, then commenting and linking. Posing questions and offering answers with reference to other bloggers are all a good way to go. As with any relationships, though, it's important to keep things rolling on with replies and the appropriate sprinkling of pleases and thank yous.

Being a reasonably anti-social creature, I'm not terribly fussed about real communities, however, I'm delighted to participate in online communities with more vigour than I do eyeball-to-eyeball ones. The reason is the off button. I don't have to have anything to do with it if I don't fancy it. Log off and the obligation goes away.

This is a big advantage, according to Terri: 'With community on the internet you can switch it off if you don't like it. You have a lot more control. You have control over your blog. That's a good thing.'

It's also community – when it suits you – that is stripped of the many things that make flesh-and-blood community less than satisfactory. There's no mess of intimacy, no confusion of mixed messages and it's quicker and more convenient. Also

Blogging for happiness

there's no cost, travel or stress about looking or sounding a certain way.

With so many of us seemingly busy beyond comfort, real community is perhaps one of the things that slips away when time is tight. We are just too rushed to attend events, phone friends or take part in activities... so isolation is inevitable. Sheila Averbuch started her blog *Stopwatch Gardener* as a side effect of ramming her passion for horticulture into the available slivers of her hectic day. She found the blog brought her much more than just an outlet for an irrepressible enthusiasm; it led a community to her: 'The blog has let me find and speak with other gardening addicts and bloggers: in fact two of my posts that got the most conversation going with readers were about gardening and about blogging itself, after a celebrity BBC radio gardener made scathing suggestions about garden blogs in general. Hell hath no fury like the blogger scorned. The BBC gardener's question time radio show later put a link to that blog post above, which sends me many new readers, so all is forgiven.

'A surprise benefit [of blogging] I had not expected is that the blog and my associated Twitter account has put me on speaking terms with celebrities in the horticulture world, like writers, broadcasters, Chelsea garden designers. We swap tips, stories, weather anxieties... they may be famous, but they put their wellies on one foot at a time, just like the rest of us.'

It's all very well being part of a jovial band of bloggers in the good times, but what about when things don't go well. How does sharing your experiences online work then?

'The thing about the negatives is the more you get them out and finish them off, the more you put them to bed so to speak,' said Terri Bodell. A problem shared is a problem halved, they say. Yeah right. A problem shared is a needy friend people avoid or a flaky colleague who can't be trusted. Unless, of course, there's another way.

Blogging about the really hard times can be hugely cathartic. My own experience of writing about both my 20-week miscarriage and the death of my brother were comforting and

How a blog can create happiness

helped 'deal with' things. Both the exercise of 'getting it out' in a post and of finding people who absolutely understood made me feel better.

In my case, typing my story out allowed me to order my thoughts and find perspective. It also, for me very importantly, let me do it in a way that didn't bore my long-suffering friends and family rigid or have me turn into the kind of emotionally incontinent victim who draws nothing but pity and discomfort. And I loathe the feeling of losing control of my emotions in public.

Even in the most orderly of existences there are times when life threatens to swamp a person. You know, something unexpected happens and it gets in the way of getting on with things. It doesn't matter how much of a cool customer you are, it isn't always possible.

Then, there are the other occasions when what you feel or think about something simply floors you. Your emotions will not be tamed or pushed into the 'not going to deal with this right now out here in front of everyone' box in your mind. It's not weakness or failure, it's just what happens to all of us when being human overtakes being successful, efficient or just plain busy.

If you're bereaved or otherwise the victim of something horrid – redundancy, cancer, divorce, that kind of thing – those around you will make allowances for a while. For a week or so, they will be kind, considerate and happy to listen. Then they get fed up, they move on. It's not that they don't care, it's just your problems don't generally dominate other people's thoughts. They've also run out of ways to say 'oh dear, that's too bad'.

They probably do care very deeply and if you beg for attention, time and compassion they'll remember what you need and give it to you. But that's not such an easy thing to do, especially when you'd rather be back to 'normal'. So you carry on in the belief that things will be fine.

Only they aren't. Stuff – thoughts, feelings and memories – find themselves looping the loop around your brain, well and truly getting in the way of your ability to get on and do.

Many of these crises – divorce or bereavement – are depressingly commonplace yet they are still an especially painful experience for everyone involved. Not only are there all the anticipated mountains of anger, loss, grief and bitterness to climb, but after a relationship breakdown it's necessary to adjust to a different view of the future – perhaps a whole new idea of who you are and what you're all about. This isn't easy and takes time.

Terri Bodell said: 'If you've got negative things inside you then you have to get them out otherwise they feel like they're going round and round and you go into what I call analysis paralysis. Analysis paralysis is where you never really get to the end of what you're thinking. Getting it out is something I advocate for all my clients. And writing it down is an excellent tool, because if it's in our mind we don't tend to be able to look at it dispassionately. The ever-decreasing spiral means you're too close to see the wood for the trees.'

Terri often gets her clients to write things down. She sees it working in two ways, firstly as the act of releasing the thoughts onto paper or screen, and also because once it's written down you can return to it later to see how things have changed.

'You can re-read and think that's a crazy way of thinking. You might think to yourself that's a really crappy day. Perhaps you thought it was the worst week of your life then, when you go back and you read all the stuff, you think it wasn't that bad after all.'

Blogging adds another dimension to the lancing effect of writing problems down and creating a record. It takes your particular problem and puts it where sympathetic and understanding people can offer support. Perhaps like counselling for those who haven't the time to join a waiting list or the money to go private.

Dave Gallson, associate national executive director of the Mood Disorders Society of Canada said: 'We believe firmly in the power of healing power of sharing one's struggles, challenges and (best of all) accomplishments and successes. As a recent comment on our Facebook page stated so accurately, "Honesty, without shame. The more people you let into your closet, the less room there will be for shame, stigma, and skeletons to exist!"

'Stigma is broken down through discussions and open dialogue. Only through communicating with others do we find acceptance and support. We have an online discussion forum with 17,000 posts from people who are sharing themselves with others. Here they find support, offer others guidance, and share their own journeys. Whether it is through blogging, writing poetry, commenting on news stories on the internet, or publishing articles in papers, promoting communications about mental illness is key to recovery and acceptance.'

A great many blogs are born in the aftermath of something large that needs to be dealt with. Something the author is compelled to write about and share with strangers. The urge to scribble – like the heart-broken letters you write but never post – runs deep.

My son was born in 1999 after a long induced labour followed by an emergency c-section. The whole experience was frightening and disorientating. At the time we lived in the Canary Islands and my entire preparation for giving birth had been to read a book that can only be described as hippyish. With the arrogance of someone who usually got her own way, I was completely convinced that I would have a natural delivery, overcome the pain and bond instantly.

Instead, after a couple of scary days I found myself being pushed at speed into an operating theatre unsure if my baby and I would live or die. It took me a long time to stop the flashbacks and to shake off the fearful feeling. Eventually, and this is before blogging was much of anything, I wrote the whole thing down and felt instantly better.

For me, like many people, the very notion of talking face-to-face with a real human being, even one whose job it is to listen, is enough to make them run very quickly screaming. As anonymous blogger *Bumbling* put it: 'The internet is a safety net for shy or indeed introverted people – and I count myself amongst their number. It's easy to talk through a keyboard, and much more difficult to do it face-to-face.'

Lack of confidence and fear of exposing vulnerability are just two of any number of reasons why you could end up feeling isolated. Kate who blogs at the splendidly named *Giggling At It All* began her blog in response to a personal tragedy: 'I started my blog at the suggestion of my mum in January 2009 and it got taken over for a while by my response to her terminal cancer diagnosis in February 2009. It helps me loads as a person who experiences depression to write it out and comments make me feel more normal and less isolated too.'

Counsellor Dale Rockell agrees. Blogging, for him, is like a form of therapy but with the added benefit of finding a sympathetic group of people to talk to. 'What these blogs are doing is allowing people to find other people who know what they're talking about and it starts a discussion. It has become easier to find people in the same boat.

'These days we quite often aren't near to family and friends because people move away for jobs and so forth. It's a way of staying in touch with people. Especially more of us are working from home which can also be isolating.

'It's a way for people to say ok I've got this situation and what they want to do is let it out somehow. But the trouble is that there's not a lot of people listening, they're too busy shouting about their own stuff too.'

To conclude, blogging can create happiness and improve your mental health as it provides a community for you to turn too, providing invaluable support, advice or just a few precious words of comfort from others when you need it the most.

Achievement and creativity

When I think of creative people, I imagine them as eccentric, long-haired and absorbed in some project that they know to be more important than the hear-and-now. Generally that's not me, is it? Sure, I 'create' during my working life – but I certainly hope corporate annual reports or newsletters about industry are not something I'm going to be remembered for.

Gradually though, I've realised that what I put in my blog is actually creative. I whip it up from nothing in the hope that it's worth someone else reading. Like a patchwork quilt, over time, it has evolved into a body of work rather than a few odd musings. I'm really rather proud of it. Thus it has become an achievement.

Do you write with your left-brain or your right? Erm. I use a keyboard most of the time (sorry!). The left side of your brain is all about logic, rational stuff, reasoning and, probably, common sense. In some respects it's the grown-up half of your grey matter. The other side is all about making things up, imagining and generally daubing multicoloured spots all over the place any which way. Or at least it seems to me.

I have spent the greater part of my grown-up life writing one way or another. You might think that it's creative, but it isn't really. Writing for newspapers and magazines is largely formulaic and what creativity there is comes in the tiniest little chunks. So, for me, blog posts allowed the freedom to write exactly what I want, in the way I want. For example, the rules I usually write by, such as using 'proper' grammar, never asserting anything without citing the source and offering a right of reply, could go out of the window. My blog, my way.

Over the years my voice has become more and more confident. I began playing it fairly safe, telling my tales from beginning to end with few quirks and twists. But then if something amused me in my head I thought 'what the heck' and blogged it. It transpires other people thought it funny too. I became more certain about what should go in. Obviously I could have been jotting these little thoughts and flights of fancy in a notebook and keeping it under my pillow, but that wouldn't have had the same effect.

So is a blog as creative as anything someone with a painter's smock and easel can come up with? It certainly seems that way. Dil Uppal, who blogs at *Skincare For Men*, said: 'Blogging has given me an outlet to be creative and write about the subjects that interest me. It's liberating being able to write whatever I want and always a pleasant bonus to hear back from those who read it.'

So, that's it then. It's about writing what you like on topics that take your fancy. Flexing those imagination muscles so they become more powerful.

Blogger Tamsin Constable of *Looking For Dragons* found her blog allowed her to rediscover the delight of a blank sheet in a way I can really relate to: 'I'm re-discovering my love of writing. Freelance writing around a young family had become a bit joyless – it was often no more than earning a living and I'd lost a bit of the joy of writing. With the blog, I'm beginning to re-discover another throwback to my pre-children life – the pleasure of writing a story.'

Hamish McFarlane, author of *Threeplay*, began his blog, called *Difficult Second Novel*, as a serious step in his literary career. It also coincided with a move from Scotland to the USA: 'The day after my 13-year civil service career ended, I started blogging. Freshly unemployed and waiting for a visa to get me from Scotland to the United States, I sat at my dining room table and (in-between posting photos of garden squirrels) I wrote about passion instead of policy. It was a refreshing change of pace. I wanted blogging to keep me focused at a time of great uncertainty, at a time of quitting my job and selling my home, when I had the terrifying, pure choice of doing anything. And I wanted blogging to help me write a novel, a side-job I'd put off for 13 years.

'It has kept me writing, and working on what is perhaps just a different kind of book. I'm not a natural blogger, I don't always like to share. But disclosing my slips and triumphs has helped my perspective on what I hope is the second half of my life, because when you write this stuff down it's more funny than furious, more illumination than irritation. And when I look at America with my clear blogger eyes, that's as it should be.'

How a blog can create happiness

And blogging can be an outlet for creativity in another field... or garden. If you'll forgive the groanawful puns, one green-fingered gardenphile started a blog, called *Stopwatchgardener*, to allow another outlet for her passion. She is now harvesting the benefits of a successful and authoritative blog. Sheila Averbuch said: 'My passion for the garden is so extreme that gardening isn't enough of an outlet. I had hoped to find that outlet in writing about the garden, and I have. *Stopwatchgardener* helps get gardening out of my head and onto the page so I can focus on all the other things that also matter: family, friends, life in our village. Additionally, like any form of personal essay, the blog also lets me plumb the depths of a question or thought and move towards a conclusion which lets me release that thought, so my mind is at rest.'

A blog can be a record of achievement, a catalogue of the steps towards a goal – or away from something – if you like. The mental health charity Mind suggests that one way of tackling stress is 'at the end of each day, sit back and reflect on what you've done and what you've achieved, rather than spending time worrying about what still needs to be done'. Great advice indeed.

Knowledge gained

What have I learned from blogging over the past five years or so? I know my blog has gone up through the middle of much of what I've done in the same way a cane will support a growing tomato plant on the windowsill. For a start I've learned a lot about blogging. I know what tends to make a popular post and what doesn't. I've got my head around the nuts and blogs of some blogging platforms and I understand how to promote a blog post to attract a few readers.

Along the way other bloggers have helped. They've tipped me off about better ways of getting comments onto my blog, what some of the statistics mean and how to raise my profile. The support from the blogging community has been unflinching. I've also turned to them for wise opinions about blogging issues: how to handle PR requests, what to do about spammers and how to create a newsletter. While it certainly wasn't what I had in mind at the beginning, I have found blogland has been a virtual classroom.

I'm not talking about the tongue-in-cheek learnings from life with kids or slightly sneery discoveries at work, I mean proper skills that apply in the real world. Photography has been a blogging development. Groping my way through the early posts, I hadn't really grasped the value of a strong image. And besides, no one was reading it, right? I used a mixture of family snaps and images I reckoned didn't have copyright issue that I gathered along the way.

Then I realised that a few people were actually coming over to my blog for a look, so I thought I'd better make an effort. After all, if someone was coming to my house, I would try to pick up the rubbish from the floor and wipe up the worst of the food-related smears. I'd bung a wash on and make sure there was toilet roll, fresh coffee and biscuits. I reckon a lot of domestic sluttery can be overlooked in the face of something good to eat and drink. It works for me anyway.

So as there were people coming over, I had better make the blog look a little better. An investigation of the most inviting blogs revealed that the key was not too much clutter and nice photos. I got rid of the rather nasty WOB – white text on a black background – and started looking for better images. I ditched a colour scheme based entirely on my favourite colours of the moment – a particularly livid purple – and went for something subtler and slightly more put-together.

Here's where I learned about copyright. Other bloggers taught me that there are places where people generously make their photos available for anyone who wants to use them. Perhaps they are so pleased with the loveliness of their images they just want as many people to see them as possible, and some images are very lovely indeed. You can find photos on Flickr where those uploaded with a creative commons licence are available for you or anyone else to post on their blogs, subject to conditions. Just read what it says, there aren't any catches.

However, I found it just became easier to take my own photos. But it was always a bit hit and miss. Sometimes they were brilliant and I was chuffed and other times they were just, well, ordinary snaps. Somehow I couldn't make my camera catch what I saw with my eyes and I didn't know how to create the effect with smoke and mirrors afterwards.

So I started following blogs with excellent images and blogs run by photographers – professional and amateur – who wanted to show off their skills. If I saw a photo I loved but didn't know how they captured it, I asked. People were happy to tell me. I discovered the best places to manipulate photos without having to sell a kidney to afford the likes of Photoshop and I found out which techniques created what effects. They pointed me to sites such as Picnik.com where a great many special effects are there for free.

The array of freely available expert knowledge on blogs is astounding. Just this evening, for example, a quick check of the blogs I follow reveals how to make batik, a delicious recipe for barbeque wings, some tips for packing for a holiday and a review of a book I'd really like to read. And all of that is before I've gone looking for some specific information.

You could imagine the blogosphere to be one ginormous library where the authors are sitting beside their books ready to answer your questions and point you to their most relevant and informative chapters. It's true, most people when given a chance to talk on their favourite subject are happy to share their knowledge and expertise. And it's no coincidence that's the subject they are likely to blog about. More than that, they are thrilled to find an interested audience.

Even bloggers for whom their specialist knowledge is their fortune are usually happy to share some of the contents of their heads on the basis that you might come back with your cheque book for the full boonah another day.

Blogging for happiness

When boiled down, perhaps this is no surprise: the act of writing a blog must go with the knowledge that something written in the blog is going to be of some kind of value to readers.

I often garner valuable information about places to go and things to do from reading other bloggers' enthusiastic accounts of their lives. Over time I've found bloggers I like and whose opinions I trust, perhaps their families or circumstances are similar to mine. Their opinions mean a lot to me.

When facing a troubling time I've laid out the circumstances of my problem on the blog and found that support has flowed in freely. For example, when I was struggling with my son's Asperger's and failing to find strategies that worked, I blogged about it. Within a day the comments section was piled high with advice, but also with understanding. I learned I was neither alone nor doing all that badly, despite what I'd felt. In return, I've offered my suggestions about dealing with wakeful toddlers, punctuation, relations with PR people and what to do during the summer holidays... and that was only in the past couple of days.

There's also an array of how-to type sites and posts. For example, doing crafty things with my children brings me out in hives. I can't stand the gluey, sticky mess along the way to creating a gluey, sticky mess. Most of this aversion is because I just can't do it. No idea how. And I'm ham fisted. So a look at a site such as *Ready For Ten* where bloggers' craft videos are loaded actually relieves the itch. Not only can I watch a demonstration, but my kids can too, that way we all know what we're supposed to be doing. I'm still looking for a cure for ham fistedness though.

My friend, Fiona Russell, keen cyclist and outdoors blogger, has a few how-to sections about bike maintenance on her blog *Fionaoutdoors*. She demonstrates her knowledge and passes it on to me – a novice bike owner (or at least a bike that didn't have streamers coming out of the handles) – in a way that is helpful but also reinforces her position as wise woman of the cycle routes.

Other experts have designed their blogs as a teaching tool and place to show off their skills and specialist knowledge. E-books you can ping into your inbox and e-courses you can subscribe to all promise tips, advice and other nuggets of self improvement. Off the top of my head, I know where I could lay my hands on e-books about using Twitter, running a business, creative writing and making bread.

But the learning isn't limited to topics of special expertise. Part of the fun is joining someone as they set out to learn something or acquire a skill. When someone you follow and know discovers something, perhaps their knowledge applies to you too. This seems to be particularly true for the mummy and daddy bloggers who are learning how to deal with the new things a baby/toddler/child lobs at them on a daily basis.

And it goes both ways. There's as much value in sharing your own (excuse me while I use this phrase) learning journey. Commit yourself to reporting your progress or otherwise and it can be a huge incentive.

A quick glance through the foothills of the blogscape reveals writers who are talking about training for a sporting event, negotiating their way through the special educational needs jungle or discussing what they found on their real-life travels. So while there's much knowledge to glean and a good few learning curves to borrow by visiting blogs and talking to bloggers, the exercise of blogging can be hugely instructive. If for nothing else than improving your clarity of thought.

Perhaps the ripest area for education is self knowledge. If my blog has taught me anything, it has been more about myself. Sometimes in a busy life, notions and influences swirl around the everyday and it's terribly difficult to form coherent thoughts.

My blog has helped me solidify my ideas about being a feminist (I am), which kind of parent I am (one who isn't a 'kind'), how we view and handle the news and how important my writing is to me. It has also shown me how far I've gone in my journey, particularly from the darkest days. I occasionally look back to what I was talking about a year or two ago. It's fascinating.

Eva Cyhlarova, head of research at the Mental Health Foundation said: 'Writing down our thoughts in a blog or on paper gives us the chance to review them later and to reflect on them in a different context, for instance when we are not caught up in negative thinking; this reflection can also be very beneficial.'

So record the knowledge you have gained from bloggers and the knowledge you have shared. When you look back later on you will be amazed at what you have learnt, what you taught others and how far you have come on in your personal development.

Doing good for others

'One voice is rarely loud enough – a whole host of bloggers just might make a difference.' Susanne, *Ghostwritermummy*

It is clear bloggers have considerable muscle when it comes to raising awareness as well as funds. They are a powerful force for charities and other campaigns. Victoria Pires, who is better known as blogger *Glowstars*, supports Vision which raises funds for the benefit of blind and visually impaired children. She heads the team behind Vision's Gold Challenge Bloggers for Vision wherein fundraisers take on a number of Olympic or Paralympics sports whist raising money and she has been roping other bloggers in for support of all kinds: 'Bloggers for Vision is another way of bloggers supporting a charity. Hopefully we'll be able to have a little fun while we're at it. In terms of the charity we're another means of raising awareness and hopefully funds.

'For bloggers I'm not so sure the benefits are as clear cut. With the Gold Challenge we all hope to be getting a little fitter and for some of us the chance to try something new. It'll provide us with the opportunity to blog about what we're doing but in terms of additional traffic for our blogs, I'm not convinced it'll bring about a great deal. I guess my motivation is that I was feeling that I should do something to support a worthy cause and Vision was the first presented to me that I felt I could support and do something for.'

Tragic events can spur bloggers into action. Charity auctions have leaped into being after various disasters such as the Japanese earthquake and famine in East Africa. But these inspiring examples are a mere flea on the tail of the dog of good works that resides in the blogosphere. There are sponsored events, auctions, fun fundraisers, petitions and common-or-garden begging.

Internet experts agree that at least half of all web time is spent mooching – catching up on friends and seeing who's saying what about whom. Included in that is seeing what your pals are in to, which includes the charities and causes they care about. OK, I know there's nothing new about this. For almost as long as there have been children, there have been sponsor forms to be passed around long-suffering colleagues, friends and family.

We've long been used to seeing images of suffering in far off places. Perhaps we've even been moved enough to get our wallets out. The real success of Live Aid, then the plethora of other celeb-fuelled beg-a-thons, has been down to the tear-jerking reports by singers and comedians of what they found on their visits. A human voice tells the tale of misery and, this time, we listen. It's much more effective than the professional news reporters of the media who don't cry on screen generally.

And so it is with blogs. On the www pages writers relate the real, moving and shocking sagas of why they care enough to support one charity or issue over another. Then because you know the blogger isn't either a trained carer or someone whose job it is to professionally report in a way that removes the heat of emotion from their story, then you know what you read is 'real'.

During journalism training I learned that objectivity is all. 'The reader doesn't care what you think – if the facts are strong enough, people will be moved by them alone.' Clearly in matters of hard news, that's how it needs to be, but it is also the very reason why bloggers are so effective when they spread the word for charities. They do give emotion, genuine heart-hurting feelings, that move and effect far more than any professional reporter ever could.

This is why some charities have chosen to take bloggers with them into the heart of the problem they are trying to alleviate. Save the Children took various bloggers with them. Christine Mosler, of *Thinly Spread*, went to Mozambique and Sian To of *Mummy Tips*, Eva Keogan of *Nixdminx* and Josie George of *Sleep is for the Weak* went to Bangladesh. *Rosie Scribbles* went to Cameroon with UNICEF.

Their reports make affecting reading.

I've been mulling this over for a while. I have a constant low-grade guilty feeling that I could be doing more to improve the lot of the many people less fortunate than I am. However, I'm not a very good volunteer – I seem to have too much on and never enough spare money or time to do anything else. I try to sponsor my chums and hand over for good causes if I don't have to go too far out of my way to do so. Philanthropy is not really my strongest suit.

However, in the hunt for inspiration for this section I had a bit of a browse through my blog archives. And I realised I've posted several times on subjects close to my heart. I've tried to raise awareness and understanding of autism and I've offered support to people who have had miscarriages or depression, both of which I care deeply about. I've banged on about punctuation and good manners. And I'm finding my voice as a feminist is getting stronger. Will I make any difference with this? Who knows, but possibly, just possibly, I might shift one person's viewpoint ever so slightly in a positive direction and if that happens, it hasn't been a waste of time.

Equally if making a hoo-ha about a cause I am passionate about, or blogging about a fund-raising event that then makes a couple of folk have a look at what the fuss is all about and, even, dip their hands in their pockets for a few quid, then that's worth it too.

But, you could argue, a blogger isn't really doing anything different to someone taking their kid's sponsor form into the office or giving an interview to a reporter from the local paper. How can banging on about it online be any better?

Good question.

Dan Hughes, who blogs at *All That Comes With It*, organised a sponsored walk along Hadrian's Wall in July 2010 to raise funds for the Joseph Salmon Trust. In the end he – with the help of 50 plus walkers and dozens of helpers – were able to hand over £26,000 to the charity.

Joseph Salmon was the son of a friend of Dan's who died at the age of three. The charity was founded as a memorial to him. It supports parents who have lost a child by providing financial assistance to those who need it most. Grieving families have enough to deal with without worries about where they will find the money to say goodbye to their child or pay the next electricity bill.

This massive success of the Hadrian's Wall walk was in no small part down to blogging. Dan said: 'Bloggers tend to have extended social networks who feel invested in their lives, and also tend to be good communicators. I found that the bloggers of the party were generally able to raise more money from individual donations than non-bloggers (on the whole).'

Having a blog perhaps affords you a strong voice to explain why you're doing something and, hopefully, persuade people to join you. For example, if your blog has talked about a cause – perhaps a condition a loved one has suffered from – then your readers know the affect it has and have great sympathy for you. So when you come along with a thing they can do to help – such as supporting a fund-raising appeal – they are more than happy to do so.

Bloggers have also been fairly effective at making the world a smaller place. From laptops all over the world we can tap tap tap connections with people we'd have no chance of coming across otherwise.

'The fact that bloggers from all over the world were involved increased the media interest in what was essentially a sponsored walk for a tiny local charity. We had local newspapers from all over the world covering us – from Idaho to Amsterdam, as well as an interview on BBC Radio Leeds,' added Dan.

Bloggers make it easy for journalists to find and tell the story too. A well laid-out appeal on a blog with lots of supporting images and background information is a dream for a hard-pressed, or possibly just idle, reporter. A blog will put the human face onto a charity appeal – fill in the back story if you like. When a news desk has dozens or more charity stories jostling for position, it can be nearly impossible to pick one, particularly if you're pressed for time. So a blog that serves up the whole heart-warming/breaking (delete as applicable) tale on a plate is going to be streets ahead in the running.

But it isn't all about charity and causes. Bloggers use their little corner of the internet as their personal soap box to lay out an extensive, and in some cases persuasive, case for whatever it is they believe in.

It seems there's little bloggers can't shift when they put their collective shoulders to it. On its own, a puny blog might not seem like it can make very much difference at all, but it can. As part of a community and speaking the truth with an authentic voice, in fact, bloggers can have a great deal of impact.

How blogging can help in the real world

'While technology can help us to keep in touch, it is no replacement for face-to-face human interaction.' Eva Cyhlarova, head of research at the Mental Health Foundation

When I'm out of sorts the last thing I want to do is socialise. I become uncomfortably self conscious, tongue-tied and dull-witted. All I want to do is stay at home alone, or, at least with my family who are stuck with me, however unsparkling I am. Yet, I know I need to get out and see people because it's Good For Me.

In my difficult times, I've ignored invitations to go to weddings, concerts and tea parties. With a family, husband and job, it was really easy to slip under the social radar without anyone noticing. Then when the time came to talk to people about something other than the menu for supper, what stage the homework is at or the word count of a particular article, it's even harder to get back into the social groove.

Blogging is a marvelous outlet for the shy – ideas and witticisms just flow onto the screen in a way unimaginable in real life. But, on its own, it doesn't really take you any closer to social grace and gregarious confidence. Or does it? In fact it's hard to see how the solitary act of blogging can help restore one's talking-to-real-people mojo, but I assure you, it can.

Here's how it went for me. You know how sometimes you can't face the world and the thought of leaving your at-home-in-your-PJs cocoon makes you shudder? But then you just have to because you've made arrangements you can't get out of, too many excuses to a friend, or something that just has to be done and not getting on with it is starting to make you feel wrong and guilty.

You sort of know that when you get there and get going, it'll be fine, riding-a-bike style. You might even forget to be awkward long enough to have fun. But getting from here, at home, to there, out in the bright lights, can feel difficult to the point of impossible.

There is a moment when you hope a minor disaster will occur, a breakage or interruption, something infectious but not uncomfortable, a way of letting you off the hook with honour, but it doesn't. So you just do it, you know your friends and colleagues are going to be waiting. The pal you only usually talk to by text has put her glad rags on and is already sitting in the pub and you'll let her down if you don't go. The baby sitter is booked – you just have to do it.

So how does blogging help with all of this? As with all things that aren't easy, practice is the key. I'm not suggesting you rehearse your tinkling social laugh and all those 'wow, I'm really interested in what you're saying' comments with your blog followers – that would be a bit deranged, wouldn't it?

But social skills, like any other, need to be brushed up on, particularly if they have become a bit battered by life. And you can do that through the medium of the internet. There are the online equivalents of the after-work pint (ah, remember those days?), the mums and toddlers coffee morning, and night out with the girls or boys.

There's the Twitter party. It's kinda like a cocktail party in a fancy bar, only you'll feel welcome and not at all awkward that you don't know anyone. Also, no one will care that you've got last season's fashion on and not done your hair. There's no requirement for high-maintenance preparation or even that ungainly juggling of drink and canapé in order to shake hands.

Twitter is not strictly blogging, but for the purposes of mojo restoration I'll include it as a microblog. What happens is you find a party. Try searching for 'Twitter party'. Or watching what's trending, perhaps there's a group talking about something that fires you up. Just have a look and join in. You don't need an invite, that's the point of Twitter – if it was private it wouldn't be there.

Twitter party organisers fix a time and a hashtag – a label to enable you to find each other in the crowd of tweets – and all you have to do is be there. Turn up at your computer – or smartphone – at the appointed hour, search for the hashtag and join in... or loiter around the sides clutching your drink if you prefer.

It's a very easy way to get back into the habit of making conversation. Joining in with twit-chat gets you used to the idea that what you have to say is interesting and entertaining, talking to people can actually be fun rather than a chore or a scary thing. It'll also reinforce the notion that what you have to say is important and worth listening to. For some of us, from time to time, we lose sight of that.

And there are other routine events you can tart up your blog for, to get virtually out and about. Just to give your confidence a bit of oomf. Blogging diaries can have many regular fixtures. These are the equivalent of meeting your mate for a coffee every Tuesday morning or having Sunday lunch with your mum. A regular comforting punctuation to the week, perhaps even – in extremis – something to hang the rest of your day around.

For example, a couple of social media experts hold a weekly clinic on Twitter. They fix a time and date and establish with the use of a hashtag, a #smclinic (that is a social media clinic) and away they go. Some folk turn up with a serious question but others are just there for the virtual beer and skittles.

There's also a Twitter pub quiz or two kicking about. Ideal if you want your long-distance social interaction to feel a bit like going to the boozer and, if you've got your wits about you, you might even win. At the very least, this mental engagement will put an end to navel gazing for a while.

Try logging on to Twitter during a sporting or entertainment event to find more like-minded friends. I'm writing this in the small window of possibility that Britain's Wimbledon hopes are still alive in the form of Andy Murray. When he plays the quarter final Twitter will be awash with Andy fans giving a point by point commentary and tweets of encouragement. (Update, Andy gave a reasonable account of himself, but it wasn't good enough in the end. On Twitter there was a volley of tweets about whether or not he was good enough or even British enough.)

During nail-biting moments of excitement in the likes of reality shows *America* or *Britain's Got Talent* and *The Apprentice*, in 140 characters or fewer, brief communities are born, awash with in-depth analysis of the performances and witty comment (sometimes). Nevertheless, you need never feel lonely during a big TV moment again.

Members of the BritMums community I loiter at occasionally volunteer to host a carnival on their blog. They collect nominations and suggestions for blog posts within a certain time range or on a specific subject and edit them into one link-heavy post.

Blog events come along on a regular basis and give you something to put in your diary and a reason to communicate with the outside world. At the moment I regularly put my oar in to Feminist Friday and Silent Sunday. Silent Sunday is an excuse to post a salient photo that sums up your week. It used to be hosted by *Mocha Beanie Mummy*, but she recently stepped back from the chore, yet, Silent Sunday has captured the imagination and continues under its own steam. I contribute to and sometimes edit the Scottish Roundup of blogs that comes out on a Sunday, which fills a flaccid Saturday quite neatly.

And, through doing these, I've met some people I'm pleased to call real friends, gained some amazing opportunities and generally improved my life.

The blogs you like to read will probably feature some sort of joiny-in type event. The on-going ones I come across on a daily basis include prompts for creative writing, invitations to write open letters, an excuse for a rant, a choice of music. And don't worry about not being welcome, every new follower or participant is more power to the hosting blogger's elbow. Do take a moment to be certain you know what the rules and etiquette are and, if you don't, just ask.

By the way, these social online get-togethers aren't generated by some sort of official or professional organisation. They've just been dreamed up by a blogger who fancied getting something going that they would be at the centre of. They often get a badge gizmo designed to allow people to let the world know what they're up to. These are generally more-the-merrier free-for-all type affairs, and they're very friendly. If you're not sure, just ask someone who has a badge on their blog, they'll be more than happy to help you. We're like that, us bloggers.

Then there are ad-hoc theme posts you can join in with. There's a thing called a meme which is defined as 'an idea, behaviour or style that spreads from person to person within a culture'. If you're not sure about diving straight in, start with reading all the posts that do take part, then start commenting – talking to the participants. That way, you'll soon get a feel for how the thing works.

A blog post, especially one that sparks comment – or even fury – is a great way to get some social interaction going. Write it, post it, put it on Twitter and Facebook then sit back and wait for the talking to start. If your post reflects something topical – the latest high-profile scandal or silly name for a pop star's child – then that's even better. It's a great way to get ready for a foray into the real world.

So how does this help you face the outside world and talk to people face-to-face? Well, blogging and its siblings, tweeting and facebooking, can hold your hand and give you confidence in your ability to talk, listen, joke and empathise with others. It affirms that you are good company, that you do have things to talk about and you can be part of a conversation. I have been known to give myself a pep talk before going to an event that goes along these lines: 'Ellen, you have a lovely blog where loads of people read what you write because it is funny and interesting. If you can write funny and interesting things you must be funny and interesting – so go knock them dead!'

How to blog

Given that I remember the first time I saw a digital watch outside of a James Bond film (on the wrist of a primary school class mate whose parents spoilt him with expensive luxuries), it's no surprise that I am constantly astonished by the innovations and glitteriness of technology. Since I started writing this book, there has been a whoosh as a whole new set of breakthroughs has rushed past me. I've tried to keep up the best I can, but I have food to eat, books to read and family to spend time with. So, inevitably, I have failed. Therefore, I won't even attempt an exhaustive exploration of this digital world as it would certainly be old-hat by the time I got to the end. I have, instead, included the major organisation and sites that look to be around for a while.

Where do I start?
Your road to online hipness will probably start along the fairly well-trod path of picking a name and joining one of the major blogging platforms such as Blogger and Wordpress.

Now it is worth spending a few minutes considering what you'll call your blog. I almost certainly didn't spend long enough considering my online moniker. *In A Bundance* came to me because, and this is going to sound very peculiar, I like the way a hypnotherapist I visited many years ago used to say things were abundant. I also sniggered internally at the idea of buns – a much better word than bread rolls – cavorting around the dining table. At the time I couldn't imagine anyone actually reading my witterings so, I thought, it didn't matter much. Fortunately it's meaningless enough to apply to whatever I want to bang on about even now. And I can still hear 'abundant, abundant, abundant' in my head while the bakery items do the polka.

Knowing how easily bored I get, I knew from the beginning that I didn't want a blog that limited my options. I didn't want to join the mummy blog band by mentioning 'mummy' in the name, although I am a mummy who blogs. For me this decision was probably because blogging is a me-time activity and I therefore wanted it to be about far more than just my offspring and their antics. And when I started writing in the parent blogging world it was already busy but nothing like as hectic as it is now. I'd say it was almost impossible to imagine that there can be another permutation of blog name that includes the words 'mum', 'mummy', 'mom' or 'mother', isn't it?

So have a think about what you're going to talk about and who you'd like to read it. If you have an area of expertise that you're going to share then go with that, for improbable example, *Ellen's World Of Household Efficiency* or *How To Raise Children Who Don't Smell Bad*.

While you probably don't want to go down a literary cul-de-sac, it is often a good idea to give readers a clue of what they might expect when they click their way onto your blog. Just as book readers make a split-second decision based on the titles and covers of books at their local bookshop, whether they're headed for the pastel coloured chic-lits or the licking flames of the vampire tomes, blog readers do similar. The name of the blog – as well as the impression a first glance at the landing page make – will have a huge bearing on whether a visitor sticks around or not.

Clearly you can call your blog whatever you fancy, but try it out on your pals – or at the very least Google and tweet it – to make sure it's not going to bite you on the backside one way or another. Is it so similar to another blog, that the other blog owner will be miffed? Is it inadvertently offensive? Does it identify you in some way you don't like?

A word on irony: British people, especially, love their quirky, irreverent, aren't-we-clever jokes, but often they don't work on the internet. In the same way that the clever, jokey headlines beloved of the UK's tabloid newspapers don't translate online, beware of being too clever as people have an irritating habit of taking you literally on the internet.

So once you've given your creation a name, then it needs a home. Probably the simplest way to get going is to use one of the gigantic free blogging platforms such as Blogger or Wordpress. In a matter of moments you can set up a blog of sorts. Blogger, for example, allows you to select one of their templates and pick and choose the features your blog might have. Basically fill in the boxes and off you go! It couldn't be simpler. Don't worry too much about these choices. It's easy to change anything you like, anything, that is, apart from the blog name.

The disadvantage of going with the flow and choosing a platform like Blogger to do all the technical parts for you is that you don't have the last word in control. Should the host breakdown, vanish or decide it doesn't like what you're doing, there really isn't much you can do about it.

A salutary tale comes from a pop music blogger who had over a couple of years established a lively and influential music blog. He often showcased new releases or the best bits of unsigned bands, always with the permission of the performer. However, one day someone on the business side of a record label spotted this and didn't understand that the blogger had discussed the matter with the artist before posting his music. They, in turn, contacted the host who promptly deleted the blog due to breach of copyright. The blogger was distraught. Years of work seemed to have disappeared in a puff of nonsense.

Eventually after a bit of a campaign and some serious unraveling of the misunderstanding tangle, he got his blog content back and very quickly went off to host it himself.

Self hosting is the other main avenue. You will have to pay a domain hosting site for maintaining your site name, then you'll need some software to set it up. Some, such as Wordpress, can be downloaded for free, but the whole exercise requires a little more time and patience.

There are virtual e-shelves full of texts on the technicalities of the internet, coding, html and all manner of other geeky and mysterious things. Don't let these deter you! Getting off and going with a blog is far, far easier than, say, doing a first-time grocery shop online or trying to work out which insurance really is the best for you.

As the saying goes, I drive a car but don't need to know what's going on under the bonnet. Same thing with blogs and it's considerably easier to get rid of the L plates.

Gordon Darroch, who blogs at *Unreal Domain*, *Autistic Dad* and *Words For Press*, said: 'Blogging is something you very much learn as you go along. You begin with an empty screen and fill it bit by bit, and after a while you find the blog's developed its own momentum. That's helped by the interactive nature of blogging, which was the big novelty for me. You start getting scraps of feedback, then you get drawn into discussions below the line, or people's comments give you ideas which spin off into further blog posts. And then you start diving into Twitter and Facebook and mining other blogs for new topics and counter-arguments. Before you know it, you've become obsessed with your web traffic and you're trying every trick to pull in a couple more readers to top last month's stats. That's when you know you're a fully-fledged blogger!'

What should I write?

Be an expert, go niche, pick a topic and go with it. I've heard instructions like this all over the internet. Writers of all stripe are being instructed to concentrate on just one tiny aspect of their best subject and stick to it. If you are planning to charge vast fees for specialist consultation, write a world-changing book or embark on a blog for strictly commercial enterprise then focusing on something specific is probably for the best. But that's not where we're at here, when we're talking about blogs and improving your mental health.

To me, specialising would be like saying I'm only going to wear one style of clothes or listen to one type of music. I would be bored within days. My blog is about anything that crosses my mind and, in my opinion, needs said.

How to blog

That said, I've just started another mini blog to collect memorials. I noticed while out and about that there are loads of memorials – benches, plaques and whatnot. I always stop and read them and wonder. They were all erected in the memory of someone special. I decided they were worth collecting and so *In Memoriam* was born. As well as paying some respects, it's a little experiment in a blog with a tight format and infrequent updates.

There is an old maxim bandied about in creative writing classes that says 'write about what you know', although I'm not sure where that puts J.K. Rowling or Terry Pratchett with their vivid and fantastical creations of Hogwarts and Discworld! It certainly makes sense to stick to topics you're close to, otherwise you're either setting yourself an almost impossible task or embarking on a work of fiction. Either is fine, but not really something I can help you with.

I asked a few keen bloggers what they write about. Trish Burgess of *Mum's Gone To...* said: 'My theme is a diary of holidays we have as a family, hence the title "Mum's Gone to..." which began with our trip to Iceland.

'However, as I can't be on holiday all the time, (shame) the blog has morphed into other aspects of my life so posts can be about many things including my amateur dramatics. I'm sure this probably muddies the water as I'm neither a mummy blogger nor a travel blogger, but it keeps me happy.'

Trish's blog has evolved into something that suits her and her life. It's a common phenomenon that blogs grow with the blogger. I started out writing about food quite frequently and, while I certainly haven't lost my appetite, these days I leave that to the expert food bloggers. It wasn't a conscious decision, it just seemed to happen. Perhaps I used to express my creativity with an inventive stir-fry and now that need is being met by what I regularly cook up on the pages of my blog. That said, I could just as easily post about a meal or dish tomorrow if I thought the topic tasty enough.

At one point, I reckoned readers would be fascinated to share the progress of an extension we were having built. But it didn't take long before I realised that news about our choice of window frames or the leaky roof issues were going to raise a big fat 'so what?' and that I could barely be bothered to think about it myself, let alone write a blog post.

On the other hand, during the gestation of the extension I spent quite a long time loitering around the blogs of interior design, home style and builder type blogs, people whose enviable good style just shone out of their blogs. For example, Nomita at *Ebabee*, said: 'I blog about stylish stuff for under fives and their mums. I have only one strict rule for my blog – I will only ever write about something that I genuinely believe is stylish, cool, unique, etc.

'When I found out I was pregnant I seriously had this overwhelming fear that my home would turn into one huge pink or blue frill. So I started searching for simpler and more minimal baby stuff and I found some fab stuff. Some I bought, some I couldn't afford and some I just drooled over.

'I just then thought why not write about it. I didn't plan it, didn't think about it, not even sure I really knew what a blog was but just started it one fine day. It's an outlet for stuff I love but can't buy as I have limited space and limited funds. And I don't find myself yearning nearly as much as before because every day I find something else I want.'

Of course, such clear definition is far from essential. Sometimes life flings up a signpost that shows you a very clear direction to travel. Tilly from *Tilly Tatas* said: 'The first blog I started is a bit of a jack of all trades. I just write about what's going on in my life: sometimes it's the kids, the pets, or a holiday (not very often), knitting, quilting, family history, our attempts to grow our own veg, an occasional moan too.

'Now and again I blog about more personal stuff. I had a 'missed' miscarriage before I had [her second child] Tiddler. That was a terrible time and I think blogging helped.

'I started my second blog to chart our "journey" with [her first child] Nipper who has finally been diagnosed with autism, sensory processing disorder and a language processing problem. The whole diagnostic process has been very confusing and frustrating. I got a lot of support and information as a result of writing the blog. I hope that anyone else going through the same thing might find my blog of help.'

Tilly decided to write about Nipper's autism because she didn't think her regular readers would appreciate a 'deluge' of frustrated posts about diagnosis and health care issues. As an aside, it's interesting that she anticipated she would be frustrated to the point of deluge, but if you read many blogs of people on a similar 'journey' then you'll see it's not surprising.

Her blog is now part of a thriving autism blog community. It's a community I meander round from time to time, interested because my eldest son has Asperger's Syndrome. There have been times I've taken to Blogger to share my exasperation, fears and joys on the subject. I've found a great deal of help and comfort from 'talking' to parents in the same boat.

A decision to create a blog on something such as autism can be a reaction to the shock and pain of a diagnosis. I found that blurting out my feelings to a community that understands is a hugely beneficial experience. Like having a room full of friends ready with cheer and wise words.

I make sure my posts about my boy's condition match our household philosophy and policy about having an Aspie in the team. For us his differences are just that, simple differences, no more nor less than being left handed, having red hair or wearing glasses. He is very able and, with support, I see no reason why he can't reach his potential and have a happy time along the way, especially as we are lucky in the level of help we get locally. So, going along with that reasoning, posts about autism feature in my blog as issues arise in just the same way as posts about all the other things that decorate my life.

There is a school of thought that says there should be a different blog for each function to make things easier for readers who want posts on only one subject. I suppose you could call that the topical approach, whereas mine is a holistic blog that looks at everything that's going on for me. Either is just as valid, it just depends on what you want to do. Conceivably it's a tad arrogant to think someone will be interested in what's going on in my head/house/life, but, then again, I did set out not expecting anyone to be listening and have been vaguely surprised when they were.

Another autism mum uses her blog, not to give voice to thoughts about her child's condition, but to remember that the diagnosis of her offspring isn't all that she's about. *Aspie in the Family* said: 'Getting lost in life is a common occurrence in my life. My scattergun approach to blogging does allow me to touch on passions and infatuations that, these busy days, feel like a bit of an indulgence.'

Jennifer Howze, known to thousands as *Alpha Mummy* at *The Times*, has found her own blogging inclination changing over time. But now blogging has gone full circle and she finds she is returning to her original interests – the ones that fired up her passions before she became a parent: 'I blogged at *The Times* with *Alpha Mummy* for four years and loved the combination of topics of parenting culture, feminism, childcare issues and just the crazy world of parenting.

'When I launched [her new blog] *Jenography.net*, I'd planned on replicating that formula. Now I'm moving more back toward travel and cultural identity as topics – things I'd written about before I got in the "mummy world". I still consider myself a mum blogger but it's all mixed in with other topics now.'

Jennifer's shift in approach from the topical – with *Alpha Mummy* – to the holistic reflects what's going on in her life at the moment, as the mothering experience becomes, perhaps, less intense. Sara's blog *Walking With Angels* gets its name from her struggles to cope with the loss of a child. Her experience has undoubtedly coloured every aspect of her life, yet grief is far from the only topic on her blog menu: 'What's on my mind generally finds its way to my blog. I wonder if I should be more structured, but I guess that's not who I am.

'I blog about my grief, how I am finding life, the joys of parenting, the moments I want to strangle my kids, holidays, days out, competitions they do. I also try to raise awareness for our charity and others close to my heart.'

Sara's remarkably candid and moving accounts of her everyday life reflect the fact that her sadness will never completely go, but that with a houseful of children it weaves its way through everything, the joy, the chaos and the ordinary everyday life.

Grief seems to be the catalyst that brings many a blog to life. Blogging about loss and trauma can be a highly effective form of 'talking therapy'. Caz from *After Anabelle* said: 'I blog about my life in the aftermath of my daughter's death. She was born sleeping in June 2010. Three months after Belle died I started blogging. It was an immediate release for me, my space to "get it all out", an outlet for my grief and to process the hugeness that became life. It's been a life-line in my coping and survival strategy but I also hope that it now raises awareness of what it really means to be a bereaved parents, that stillbirth still happens and to break the silence surrounding it.

'I call it a journey blog because I guess I see it as my diary of the journey of putting my life back together. I know it will never be completely back together; there is an Anabelle-shaped hole that cannot be fixed, but already along the way I'm encountering highs, lows and lots I didn't expect as well as coming so far.' At the time of writing Caz is expecting her second child.

Allison Rosser has a blog called *Cancer And Baby Equals Chaos*: 'I blog about our journey through life since my fiancé was diagnosed with cancer a week before our third child was born. Life has changed a lot for us during my time as a blogger and I have tried to emphasise that with my blog.'

It's that word 'journey' once more. It keeps coming up again and again. So to stretch that metaphor, whatever direction that travel is going in, a blog provides an excellent record of the miles covered and sights on the way.

Arguably any blog that details the progress of everyday life is a journey of sorts. A glance back over the pages of my blog gives me a view of how things have changed over the years. I know it's a fairly navel-gazey exercise, but an interesting one nonetheless – sort of like the marks on the kitchen wall logging my kids' growth.

Many of the hundreds of blogs that burst into life every day are conceived in the owner's passion – whatever that might be. Tamsin Constable started her wonderfully named blog *Looking for Dragons* to explore the natural world and get outdoors with children: 'I keep *Looking for Dragons* loosely focused on wildlife/ adventure/ outdoors, because that's what I've been interested in since my own childhood. I think of myself as a writer who wants to explore Yorkshire and the natural world (often with my children because they happen to be around a lot!), and communicate this to a wider audience (there's a bigger underlying agenda, of course, about environmental issues and fighting an over-protective culture).'

Many passionate bloggers take it up because their enthusiasm for whatever their thing, is it is too great to be absorbed by the mere thing alone – and they need to write about it too. Is that how it is when a hobby spills over into obsession? If so, then a passion blog isn't just an outlet, it's a public service. Golf fanatics, perpetual knitters, sports car enthusiasts and trashy telly addicts can share their love without boring the knickers off their nearest and dearest.

Actually that is flippant, but if you don't have much of an interest in baseball, insect collecting or archaeology then you'll probably find yourself fed up fairly fast when you venture into specialist blogs on those subjects.

Talking about specialist subjects, it's almost certain that your nearest and dearest will fall into that category one way or another. Why not use it to absorb your enthusiasm for your family? Many a blog is created as a place to preserve memories and landmarks as well as a way of letting far-flung friends and relatives see the kids' progress.

Cass Baillie who blogs at *Frugalfamily* said: 'I blog about my family's life to record all of our memories in one place and even though I know a lot of people don't like the term "mummy blogger", I do think that I am one.

'One day, I'm going to print all of my posts out and have them made into a book for the children so they can look back at their childhood and remember the special moments.

'I always have in the back of my mind the reason that I blog and my eight year old especially loves to read back through it and look at photos of things we've done together. She often tells me that she thinks she's the luckiest girl in her class because we do so much together but I think that's more because of the fact that she can look through the blog at things we've done rather than us spending more time with her than her friends' parents.'

That's a fantastic idea. I know my older children are always hungry for stories about their babyhoods.

So does this all help? Do you now know what should you blog about? As you can see, it can be absolutely anything that you fancy. Something you love, hate or are learning about, it doesn't really matter. What's important is that you want to tell the world about it. I never have any problem settling on a topic to post about. It is whatever is burning a hole in my brain at any point. And the longer I do it, the more clear it is to me which thing I have to put onto a blog page first.

How do I get followers?
The quick – if somewhat glib – answer is that if you give good content, people will want to read it. That's all very well but if no one knows that your gems are sitting there, glistening all by themselves, they won't come by to admire them, will they?

So how do you get people to read your blog and come back every time you post something new? You can start by making relevant comment on the blogs you enjoy and admire. Those blog owners will see your comment, be curious about you and go to have a look at your blog. Do this as widely and as generously as you can.

Few bloggers can resist responding to a comment that says something along the lines of 'I've just found your site and I really enjoy the way you write. I'll look out for future posts'.

If you are inspired, informed or charmed by a post on someone else's blog then do them a favour by sharing it. Post the link on Twitter or Facebook, tell your friends. A grateful blogger may be more inclined to reciprocate and pass on your best offerings to their followers.

Join the gang. Or, in fact, as many gangs as you want. All over the internet there are groups, forums and networks of like-minded bloggers talking and looking at each other's content. Find one that suits you and join up. Don't just sign in and stand on the sidelines though, take part. Read what other people are saying and chip in with your thoughts, even if you are just agreeing and haven't got anything particular to add. Many of these bases have places where you can post your news or updates. Tell the world what you've just written about, that's what these places are there for.

Do a little networking. Twitter and Facebook are your friends when it comes to promoting your latest offering. Tell your Twitter followers what you've written about – and not just once – do it several times. Facebook users probably only need it once, but do post the link to your blog to your Facebook followers. Don't be bashful about this, if someone doesn't like it, they can either ignore you or, if you've really got up their noses, stop following or 'friending' you. There's nothing to stop you emailing your friends and contacts with your latest work, especially if you think it'll be of interest.

Adrian Doherty who blogs at *Earthy Android* isn't so keen on following blogs but instead follows networks and the individuals within them: 'Don't follow blogs myself, so don't expect others to. I follow people and organisations instead via social media channels.

'I promote via Google+, Facebook and Twitter but am considering adding a StumbleUpon layer given its growing popularity and semi-viral nature. I have these all tied together via Klout too ...'

In real life there are coffee mornings, dinner parties or introductions over a post-work pint. There are workshops, think tanks, conferences and seminars. You could attend a panel session, an introductory meeting or simply set out your stall in the middle of the high street. Online, it is only slightly different. You can find round ups (where one editor collates blog posts that they have either found or are recommended), linkys (like an internet conga – simply join in by pinning your post to a notice board), memes (posts on a theme that link to each other). These are as varied as their real-life counterparts. Some are formal, regular and bound by rules and others are easy-going and of the let's-do-the-song-right-here variety. And such is the wonder of the brave new digital world, that if you can't find any you like then you can set them up yourself.

For a while I wrote a few posts about miscarriage and invited other bloggers to share their experiences. Using a linky – a third-party widget embedded into the post to allow them to easily link to their sites – I hosted a few other bloggers who were talking about similar things.

Give a blog a bad name... or a good one. For a while SEO (search engine optimisation) was the hot new form of witchcraft that would bring readers flocking to your bit of the internet. This is the inexact science of working the mysterious calculations used by the likes of Google to deliver results in response to a search. Current thinking is that whatever the main topic of your post is, it should be in the title, therefore most likely to lead people searching the topic to it. For example, if you have written, say, about free climbing in the Alps then say so in the title: 'Free climbing routes in the Alps'.

It's possible to improve the likelihood of being discovered by someone using a search engine by making sure you use the subject of your post in the title and again in the first couple of paragraphs. Imagine search engines are well-intentioned but not very bright visitors and put up as many signposts and clear directions as you can manage.

After we bloggers have published a post, we will most likely engage in a little pimping – which is internet speak for letting the world know about our marvelous and compelling new offering. Obviously your followers will know there's something new to read, but most bloggers want to get more new people interested with each post. Here are the things I do with some posts:

- Put the post on Ping-o-matic;
- Put it on my Facebook page;
- Put it on the pages of other Facebook groups I think might be interested;
- Tweet it several times over 24 hours. I try to use a message that I hope will entice people to click through and read;
- I post the link onto any forums that might care.

However, that's only the few things I, with my short attention span, find work for me. If you have more energy and patience than me you could try the following: making sure your blog posts turn up on Linked-In, figuring out how Google+ works and adding 'like' buttons to the bottom of each. You can also get involved with Blip, Google Buzz, Del.icio.us, Digg and Reddit if you fancy.

Technical tips and design ideas
While content is, as they say, king, how your blog looks is important too. Once again, a stroll around the blogosphere will reveal a huge range of looks and styles. What do you like and what makes you shudder?

I'm not suggesting you copy someone else's blog design, but you can acquire a feel for the kind of thing you are after – or at least be certain about what you don't like. My blog is not of a particularly inspiring design, but I have attempted to keep it clean, uncluttered and fairly easy to look at.

Some blogs have the feel of walking into the bedroom of an over-indulged and possibly colour-blind eight-year-old girl with delusions of royalty. If that's your bag, fantastic! However, I find the flashing gif images and garish colours make me reach for my sunglasses.

Just as you will probably pause in front of your wardrobe and think 'am I going nautical but nice today, or city safari, or channelling my inner Grace Kelly?' stop and try to make your blog look a bit put-together. Chaps – it would be a bit like wearing all your best stuff (baseball cap, sandals, socks, leather jacket, designer suit, f-f-f-funky waistcoat and golf gloves) all at the same time. Too much. And, unless you know about design and stuff, make the background lighter than the text otherwise you'll give me a headache. Then I won't come back to your blog and neither will anyone else probably.

I spent a good chunk of my career working in tabloid newspapers. British tabloids are brilliant examples of how to get readers into the page and keep them there. For me, a great many of the same principals apply to blogs.

Headlines are snappy and enticing – perhaps they post a question or offer a revelation that will be answered in the text. For example, how to sustain a sex life after children, or five ways to look younger without resorting to surgery.

Big blocky chunks of text are not tempting to anyone, particularly a busy person browsing by on the hunt for amusement. Use sub headings, bullet points, pictures or any other device that chops things up into more digestible units. Don't make people work for what you're telling them because, generally, they won't bother. And in the same way make sure references and links are all there to be had – the more helpful you are to your reader, the more they'll stick around or come back for second helpings of your wisdom.

Much as a sofa doesn't look right without scatter cushions and a plate of food often needs something green on it, there are things I'd expect to see on a blog. That said, the whole point of blogging is to suit yourself so feel free to ignore or, even, violently disagree. In fact, blog about it, it'll create some cracking traffic for us both.

A blog must be updated regularly – not frequently, but regularly. Even if it's only once a month, it still needs to be consistent. A neglected blog is a sad old thing so if you decide your blog's time is up, put it out of its misery with the delete button. More posts isn't always better, you can have too much of a good thing. But find out how often you are comfortable posting and, in the main, stick with it. I aim for three times a week plus a bonus photo at the weekend.

A blog must have some means for readers to track new posts. There should be a way of signing up or following. You could use an email sign-up or an RSS (really simple syndication) link to allow new posts to be automatically sent to someone's inbox. I know these sound complicated, but I can work them so they can't be. A blogging platform such as Wordpress, Typepad or Blogger will walk you through step-by-step. Honest.

There should be somewhere for people to comment. It's not compulsory, but, for me, the ability to have a conversation is pretty important. But once again, having made your point, you might actually just want to draw a line there with the last word. In that case, turn off the comments for that post.

Pictures should be pretty. I suppose this is something to do with that saying 'if a job's worth doing, it's worth doing well'. So I'm going to assume that you want your blog to be as fabulous as possible. Perhaps you've had this poetry brewing inside you for years and the stream of verse that is spewing onto your screen is breathtaking, magnificent and rhymes too. Then don't let it down by bunging up a dreadful image with it – or, worse still, leaving it unadorned. Of course, there are gorgeous design-led blogs that use elegant fonts, graphics and white space to gasp-inducing effect, however, if that's what you're up to, you're in the wrong chapter so move along now. For the rest of us, a good picture can make all the difference. They make a page – digital or otherwise – a much more comfortable place to be. Your pictures don't have to be professional quality, just something to make the whole thing more interesting. Imagine reading a newspaper with no photos – you'd have to be a very, very keen newshound to put up with that. You can also find images elsewhere on the web – just make sure they are available for you to use without breaking someone's copyright. Try Flickr creative commons.

A blog should have links to other good places on the internet, because it is part of a web or mesh of a greater internet community. Obviously, it's perfectly possible to bumble along in isolation but the chances are not too many people will find your masterpieces and if they do, they'll find them too sterile to hang around. It would be like the friend who, every time you meet, always seems to want to talk about themselves without listening to any of your news. So links. Do you look puzzled here? It's the bit of differently coloured text where you click and are transported off to another page – kind of like something Harry Potter and his chums did in fireplaces. If you refer to something or someone and it has a page, link to it. Make it easy for people to find out what you're talking about. If somebody – perhaps another blogger – inspired a post, give 'em some link love. Not only is it helpful to your readers and good manners, but it improves all manner of statistics and rankings, should you care about these things.

You may want to consider a blog roll, which is a list somewhere on your main page of other bloggers you follow or that perhaps you think are similar to you or that your reader may like. It could be someone you're supporting by hauling their neophyte blog into the bright glare of your success (obviously). Once again, it's all about being a 'well-rounded' blogger who reads and is generous with recommendations. Old blogging timer that I am, I can now tell quite a lot about a blog from what's in the blog roll. Conversely, I've stumbled on some gems by seeing what my current blog crush's preferred reading is. I also have a huge soft spot for the seemingly humble blog roll, because more than twice I have been chuffed to be offered writing jobs because someone found my blog by trawling someone else's blog roll.

Have a means of getting in touch with you. I'm not suggesting that you go about putting your address and phone number all over the internet for every peeping, drooling Tom, Dick or Harry to find, but, once again, it's about being real and available to your readers. It's disconcerting to find a blog that has no sense of where the writer really is. There are some celebrated cases of fake blogs being written by someone entirely different to who you'd suppose. I'd suggest putting an email address (not your work or family one – unless you're very sure) on your biog bit and include a link to, at least, Twitter. If readers like your blog, then they like you and might want to talk to you. I'd say, if you take some basic precautions, there's nothing to be scared of. Yes, you might get some messages that aren't necessarily the nicest, but it's fairly unusual. And that's what the delete button is for. It's perfectly possible to be available but mysterious and anonymous too.

This is what young folk would call a 'no-brainer' – a blog must have original content. It's your place so it should be filled with your stuff not someone else's. Manners again. Don't nick things that don't belong to you, it's just not cricket. By all means discuss what others say (but link to them), be inspired or infuriated but reference it. And if something is so marvelous you must have it, just ask. A great many bloggers would be flattered and happy to be reproduced somewhere else provided they get the appropriate thanks and signposting back. Same goes for photos, videos and audio – please check it's OK to use. Analogy: if someone helps themselves to your beautiful – and abundant – crop of roses without asking you'll be pretty miffed. If they tell you how divine they are and then ask if they can have a few while promising to tell their friends where they got them, then you'll probably have a glow of horticultural smugness about you. Manners again, really.

Statistics and rankings

Lies, damn lies and statistics. Yes, we all know statistics can be massaged to say pretty much anything. However, they can provide all manner of diverting nuggets of information that can, theoretically, be used to inform the work you do in the future.

Where do they come from these magic numbers? Major blogging platforms usually have a statistics function somewhere in the back room. Have a poke around – it's normally fairly easy to find.

Google Analytics is another source of blog measurement. Once you sign up to the analytics section of Google, you'll find a piece of code that you need to post to your blog before your figures can be magically revealed.

So what do they reveal? They will tell you how many unique visitors have arrived at your blog, what they looked at and how long they stayed. They will also tell you the source – did they click through from another blog, from Twitter, Facebook or elsewhere. You can also find out which search terms they used to find your posts.

There are third-party organisations such as Technorati that produce ratings and rankings for blogs. There is some satisfaction in seeing what your position in their league tables is, however, they shouldn't be taken too seriously.

In the hands of a reasonable blogger, statistics are a useful guide to what works and what doesn't. They can tell which of your posts are most popular and which topics people wanted to read about. However, they come with a huge warning. DO NOT PAY TOO MUCH ATTENTION TO YOUR STATISTICS. A great many bloggers discover their statistics and then become obsessed by them. Certainly it's flattering and gratifying to realise that all over the world nameless readers are clicketyclicking their way onto your pages, but it's really important to remember to blog for the people who read your posts, not the counting machines that measure them.

Will you tell a stranger how much you weigh or what's in your bank account? No, probably not. And blog statistics have the same kudos. All over the internet confident and experienced bloggers are cagey about revealing how many people visit their blogs. Are we all under the illusion that everyone else has thousands of readers to your several dozen? Perhaps. What it does tell me is that the same weight of hokum around making money and losing weight is rapidly building up around increasing blog traffic and website statistics.

Are rankings rank? There are some who would say that starting to watch your progress up – or down – a rankings list is a shortcut to madness. Er, what's that? You don't know what rankings are? Well they're calculations done using metrics and, of course, some algorithms. Yup. Geeky stuff, but, at heart, anything done on computer and the internet can be measured with a bit of string – or several bits of string actually.

Rankings are basically the table tennis ladder of the internet only without the transparency or lost balls. They work on complex measurements that I have no intention of trying to understand, because they'd only go and change the next week. These formulae aren't anything like as straightforward as the number of people who 'like' or read or comment on your blog, but that does come into it. They are a measurement of influence, frequency of posts and type of content. Who links to you and how often? Are you talked about and re-tweeted? See, I told you it was fiddly stuff.

Wikio is a news portal that produces a blog ranking every month in different categories from knitting to football. Other measures can be gathered at Technorati, Klout and Peer-Index, and more seem to pop up – or I discover them – all the time. Who knows what'll be out there by the time you read this? If it's your bag, have a look at blogs in your field, ones you admire or aspire to and see what's on their pages. If they're setting the heather alight, or even slightly smouldering they will likely have a badge somewhere on their blog's front page bragging about where they rank well.

Sectors and specialisms have their own rankings or other areas of competition. For example, the Tots100 ranks parents

How to blog

who blog. At the moment what mums and dads write in their blogs is intensely important to the marking and advertising of brands aimed at families. It's a bit of a new thing and will presumably calm down when the band wagon has rumbled on to the next new thing.

Meantime it is as commercially useful for people with things to sell to know which blogs are influential as it is personally satisfying to the blogger. Of the thousands of parent blogs, Tots 100 lists the ones their magic incantations consider to have the most oomph in order. Even for those of us who don't care.

The list was started by freelance journalist and PR Sally Whittle who blogs at *Who's The Mummy?* – She said: 'When I started the Tots100 there was no single, publicly accessible list of UK parent bloggers. Finding blogs was a matter of endlessly clicking on links on blog rolls and Twitter, or googling, or paying for a list. This was a big problem for people like me who wanted to read lots of blogs but also a problem for my clients, who wanted to talk to Mummy and Daddy bloggers, but just didn't know where to find them.

'And of course, once you find a blog, it's almost impossible to tell just by looking if this blog is popular, or influential or suitable for your campaign. The Tots100 was therefore created as a place where blogs could be listed in one place, and you could easily see who was currently the most influential, popular and engaging.

'We work very hard to ensure bloggers in the Tots100 have a rewarding experience and being listed is worth their while. For starters, we try to use the site to promote blogs and help them gain new readers – by publishing our top 100 each month but also doing a weekly round-up of our 10 favourite posts from across the whole Tots100, and a monthly introduction to 12 brand new blogs alongside blog hops, which can generate traffic and also give bloggers the opportunity to win great prizes.'

Did I say I didn't care? Well just so you know, this summer I was at position 101 in the Tots 100 – about as also-ran as you can get, but this month I'm at 66.

Maggy Woodley who blogs at *Red Ted Art* is not also-ran. She's at number one in the rankings and is often there or thereabouts. Her blog's tag line is 'bringing art and colour to children's hearts'. She said: 'Being in the Tots100 rankings does drive new traffic to my site – which is always good. And of course I do mention it when I speak to potential advertisers – so I guess it provides me with "general kudos" and anyone looking to work with me is reassured that my site is half decent.'

Naturally other fields have their own listings. If you find a blogger you like and their blog has a badge saying they're part of a group or ranking, follow your nose and you'll likely find the list you want.

Competitions and awards

'If winning isn't everything, why do they keep score?' Vince Lombardi

I don't much like competition – or at least ones that I'm not sure of winning. I hate competitive sports, can't see the point of gambling, am scared by popularity contests and don't even like crazy golf or ten pin bowling. You see, for a non-competitive person, I hate losing.

What's that got to do with blogs? Isn't the blogosphere, like the second coming of the Summer of Love, all peace, harmony and cool dudes? We're supposed to be sitting around our virtual campfires typing up a crowd-sourced version of Kum By Ya, aren't we?

It's true, there is a lot of support and compassion out there, far more than, in my opinion, the face-to-face world offers. But people don't seem to be able to stop measuring themselves against each other. Perhaps that's a curse of the human condition. So if you've got a blog – you've polished it, honed it, posted on it, pimped it and generally feel quite pleased with it, then there are dozens and dozens of places you can go looking for a best in class certificate or you can find a top 10, 20 or 100 to enter.

Have a search for blog competition and you'll probably find one. There. That was simple, wasn't it?

Of course there's far more to it than that. There are competitions, there are ranking lists that work on cold hard statistics, there are events where you win *X-Factor*-style by public vote and there are awards for everything from prettiness to sharp writing.

A great many newspapers and magazines have taken to holding blogging awards, step forward *Cosmopolitan*, *The Guardian*, *Metro* et al. You could argue that it's a cynical attempt by the publication to get more website traffic... surely not. But they're in business and few things any commercial organisation does are for anyone's benefit but the owners, and shareholders, in the long run.

What these contests do is raise the profile of those involved. And, generally, it means the blog pitch is a level playing field. In theory, your musings could be shortlisted and given the same amount of exposure as one of the giants. It's possible to get your writing in – or at least in the vicinity of – a newspaper without being at the whim of whichever disgruntled subeditor is in charge of the letters page on a given day. (I know, I have in a previous life been that subeditor.)

Many contests work on a public vote system which means that you have to work for your prize. Once a blog finds itself shortlisted – whether by nominations or by the organisers – it then falls upon the entrant to put themselves about, promote and generally grovel for votes. This kind of contest makes a lot of sense to an organiser because not only do they have very little work to do and no nasty decisions, but the ensuing campaigns will guarantee all-important traffic to their sites.

Understandably, they are a very popular way of doing things at least for the organisers, but not one that I've got a lot of time for. Primarily because they are time consuming and, basically, a popularity contest not really anything much to do with the content of the blog. After all, what's in it for a reader to vote if they aren't already on your Christmas card list? That's all very well if you've got lots of followers and chums and you don't mind badgering them into voting for you, but it's not my thing.

Many participants do say they can be great fun and a good excuse for a get together and will drive a bit more traffic to a blog. In some cases they result in a real-life actual awards ceremony which, if nothing else, is an excuse to get your glad rags on.

Every community, it seems, has awards of their own. There are Canadian, Welsh and Scottish awards, prizes for political blogs of every colour, foodies, movie fans, sci-fi and science. The process of writing this section has led me to find lots of blog fields previously unexplored. Fascinating stuff and I can safely say blogging award listings can lead you to some exciting new online discoveries. And, in this case, wasted a couple of days reading when I should have been writing.

Many of the contests do work on merit alone or that merit has a part in them. There are almost as many formats as there are bloggers with the competitive instinct. Some will be shortlisted by a panel of judges, others nominated by the public then shortlisted by a panel, some voted the public to a shortlist then voted by a judge, and so on.

So whether you decide that competition is healthy or more hassle than is worth, I would suggest that you take the time to discover how it works, what effort it is going to take and what you expect to get from it. There is little more dismal than someone entering a contest then looking like a no-hoper who didn't get off the start line. Plan your strategy – how are you going to execute your campaign? Do you have readers who will be happy to support your appeals for votes (or whatever) or do you think they'd be cheesed off and you embarrassed by the whole thing? Would you be happy to be featured in your local newspaper – if it came to that – or does that make your toes curl?

On the other hand, your blog – or at least its content – can do nicely in other competitions. Do you write fiction or take fabulous photos? There are contests for them too. I entered a writing competition run by the website of STV – our local independent TV station – and was thrilled to be short listed with a blog post I'd written previously. All I had to do to enter was send them a sample of writing. The prize was a short paid contract to write opinion pieces for the website. I didn't come first in the competition but I did make contact with lots of lovely people at STV's website and I now work there regularly. So, in a way, what I did was much more useful.

There is just a word of warning – competitions can hoover up all your time, energy and hope. Pick and choose carefully what you'll enter and then take a long hard – realistic – look at what it's all about.

The blogging Oscars – the Weblog awards or Webbies – do round ups of the best blogs from all over the world into categories that include geographical region and topic. Some would say this is the original and best blogging award.

So competition, is it healthy? It all depends. It's very difficult to measure one blog against another – one might be funny while another makes you cry. And is bigger always better? There are gems of writing and insight tucked away in the back pocket of someone who doesn't care very much about promoting him or herself. Meanwhile, more gregarious bloggers are ubiquitous and that might not always reflect the quality of content. And, in any case, one person's art is another's pompous rant.

Liz Jarvis who owns *The Mum Blog* said: 'In my day job I'm currently recommending bloggers to work with professionals and I can tell you categorically that it matters not a jot to me whether they've won this award or that award or they're featured in this chart or that chart.'

Her take is that blogging is as competitive as any blogger chooses to make it. She added: 'When I first started blogging I didn't have a clue about any charts, I wasn't even a member of BritMums, d'oh. When I discovered charts my natural desire to do well in them (not least because I was blogging professionally) took over for a while, just as when working on magazines I cared about circulation.

Blogging for happiness

'Once I got over that, and took a step back, I realised I was happy to blog for myself. Now I may tweet about being in Wikio or whatever, but really, I don't take it at all seriously and I don't think anyone else should either; I check my stats maybe once a week to see what's working and what isn't but I'm never going to cry myself to sleep about not being in this chart or that chart. Some of my closest blogging friends are some of Britain's best known bloggers, and I feel so happy for them whenever they achieve anything, we all celebrate for each other.'

Liz and some of the, ahem, senior bloggers, among whom I must count myself have gone through what can only be called the blog life-cycle. Susanna Scott of *A Modern Mother*, agreed: 'I think you go in phases. There is a lovely phase in the beginning where you don't get sucked into it. Then you do. Then you come out the other end in a Zen state, not really caring, comparing and back to basics. At least that is how it was for me.'

The moral of the story is not to care too much and, if you can't manage that, don't enter the competitions and look at your statistics. It's only a blog after all.

There is a popular notion that a blogger is doing it only for themselves. On the face of it, it's hard to argue with that as, really, in most cases it's hardly an act of philanthropy. It's laughable to think you'd say: 'Today I'm going to change the world by telling everyone how I prefer to make cheesecake.'

For me certainly, I've never managed to get my cheesecake to set.

But whatever the motive, it's safe to say we want our blogs to be liked – loved even. Otherwise, why bother? How stomach churning would it be for someone to comment on your blog to the effect that they stopped by, had a look and found the content to be dull, poor, average at best and won't be back? We all have a blog-ego, a notion that something we have to say or share – or even the way in which we do it – is got to be worth someone you haven't met spending some time on.

So does my bum look big in this? Oh, sorry, wrong question. Same question actually: Is my blog any good? Do you like it?

Entering a competition can give you an answer to this. Or at least one that's more honest than the opinion of your husband/wife/mother/best pal. It might, on the other hand, give you the answer you don't want to hear: Yup, it looks huge and really rather lumpy.

Remaining anonymous
'The more people you let into your closet, the less room there will be for shame, stigma, and skeletons to exist.' Mood Disorders Canada

Do you keep secrets? Is it something about yourself, something the person sitting next to you at work or on the sofa doesn't know? Things you can't tell have a habit of making their presence felt in your mind, don't they? I find they march around my head begging to get out. Maybe I could silence them if I told someone, somehow. OK, I can't turn round now and say 'guess what?', but perhaps I could blog...

It's good to talk, according to the maxim, but you need to pick and choose the place and the people carefully or it may not be good at all. Have you ever had the experience that you reveal something, blurt out a feeling, share a view and then there's that moment when the people round about you go quiet? That's the instant you know you shouldn't have opened your mouth. Your friends edge away, the social bubble is burst and you can't do anything to fix it.

What about if you realise that the person in the supermarket knows your deep, dark secret? Yes, her over there with the green jacket. Don't look now, she'll see. And before you know it you're hiding in the pet food aisle hoping she hasn't got a cat, because you can't stand that she knows something about you that you wished you'd kept to yourself.

Online it's not like that. Whatever you share, you'll find someone who understands, relates and, often, wants to let you know they care. And there is really very little chance of bumping into them while you do your weekly shop.

Blogging for happiness

I've always found it difficult to open up. The shock, or, what's worse, sympathy on the face of a confidante is especially uncomfortable. I'm a jolly, cheery, coping kind of person to the core. In the main, it's how I am and it's certainly how I like to present myself to the world. So when the wheels came off my wagon a couple of years ago, it was terribly difficult to deal with it all revolving in my head. It doesn't help that I'm a paid up member of the Stiff Upper Lip Party – I hate blubbing in public. Tears, snot and gasping sobs are only ever behind a closed door, on my own. And even then I still feel faintly embarrassed.

But the urge to share goes deep... so I blogged. I told the world about the moment the ultrasound found my baby didn't have a heartbeat, I talked about the loss of my brother, my dad and the resultant depression that swamped me. And the good people of the blog world were able to give me exactly what I needed, someone to listen, offer a word... the written equivalent of a pat on the arm... and let me know they understood. Therapy indeed.

I decided that I would tell those stories in public – or as public as my modest blog is. Anyone with the notion, nothing better to do and a day or two can probably glue together the entire story of my recent life from what I've written on the internet. But I can't imagine why anyone would, unless they were searching for an insomnia solution or trying to pinpoint the exact moment a life becomes more ordinary.

I'm also grown up enough and settled in both my work and private life to be unlikely affected by anyone's reaction to what I've said. After a few years in the media you get a feel for what's going to rattle cages and I don't think my minuscule revelations would do that. After all, they were catastrophes of the very commonplace variety. So the revelation that I had, gasp, a mental health problem won't shock people, I see it more as, at best, a battle scar.

However, just because your story is as unremarkable as rain drops, it doesn't mean that what you have to say might not cause ripples in your own personal pond.

It may be that the issue that's burning its way out of you relates to someone close, someone who reads your own blog. How can you talk honestly about your husband or mother-in-law there? What happens if you need to reveal abuse or other criminal activity? If blogging is your therapy then you need somewhere else to go.

Luckily there are other options if your beans are screaming to be spilt. There are shared blogs that allow bloggers to write under a pseudonym, such as Blogonymous, which is a safe place for people to post without their identities being revealed. Explaining how it works, one of the group said: 'There are six bloggers that form the Blognonymous panel. As a group of like-minded bloggers, we started thinking about how we could support people who wanted advice, support or even just to vent in an anonymous fashion.

'Our research brought us to a collective of blogs, all sharing the same ideology, and we have decided to open our blogs to those who needed them.

'We decided to use our own blogs – rather than set up a brand new blog – because we had the readership established and we felt that readers would feel more comfortable commenting on something within a blog that they already knew.'

The Blogonymous team are Nickie, who blogs at *Typecast*, Paula Battle of *Battling On*, Jay of *Mocha Beanie Mummy*, Emily of *Mummy Limited*, Sandy Calico of *Baby Baby* and *Parent Confidential*, and the owner of *Bumbling's Blog* who is herself anonymous.

Explaining what motivated them to help people speak out privately, the Blogonymous spokeswoman revealed why bloggers come to them: 'Because people build up a relationship with their blog readers and sometimes need to step away from that or, indeed they want to be able to speak freely without their family and friends or work colleagues knowing who they are. Also, some people are very protective about what information they give out on the internet.'

What the women have set up is a system whereby someone with a story to tell chooses to contact one of them either by one of their blogs or by the Blogonymous Facebook or Twitter page. They email their story and it's published. 'They retain complete anonymity and, whilst we are not agony aunts or advisors, we build up a relationship with the service user. When we publish the post we often provide links to external resources, more to assist another reader who may be experiencing something similar but can't or won't speak out for whatever reason.

'Many people often need impartial advice regarding something in their life and can only obtain that by asking someone who doesn't know them personally.'

The blogonymous posts make heart-rending reading and it's easy to see why dozens of comments offer support and advice to each. Big issue topics covered include relationship breakdown, redundancy, addiction, childhood sexual abuse and children who are bullied. Some are looking for advice and others for a place to talk away from prying eyes. Others simply want to get it off their chests and, perhaps, help someone else in so doing. There is also, what I'm going to call the blog effect, where the process of transferring a mush of ideas into a coherent post helps clarify even the muddiest of thoughts.

Blogonymous has grown from merely an outlet for people to express themselves to something of a support network. As each person has come forward with a story to tell, the breadth of resources has grown: 'We find people are so willing to give up a few minutes of their time to read and offer advice or reveal their own experiences. We are building a support network of sorts – one that has no barriers and one that is neutral in the community that we hope anyone feels they can use.'

The anonymous one of the six, Bumbling, used Blogonymous, to get a few things off her chest. She said: 'I had a tough year last year, and my marriage broke down. I actually wrote a Blognonymous post before that happened, about some difficulties I was having living with a partner with depression.

'My ex-husband knew I blogged and I didn't want him to read it. Perhaps, in retrospect, I should have let him. But it was very cathartic at the time, as it was a topic I wasn't really able to talk to people in real life about, and I picked up a lot of lines of support in that way.'

Bumbling, who is a lawyer in the real world, didn't really hesitate before deciding to keep her blog life and her work one separate. She writes beautifully at *Bumbling's Blog* about her life with daughter Moo. She said: 'To be honest, it was because I was embarrassed. None of my friends blog, or do anything online other than Facebook. I wasn't sure if I'd be any good at it and thought they'd all think I was a big geek. They do anyway.

'Also, I'm a lawyer and am conscious of the fact that my online reputation would affect my professional reputation. I wasn't planning on doing or saying anything that I wouldn't under my real name, but I wasn't entirely keen on having people Google my real name looking for lawyer me and finding mummy me. Finally, I wanted to be able to avoid giving too much personal information about Moo away, although I do use her photo. A lot.'

It's interesting that she wanted to put distance between her work persona and the online mummy. It would be marvelous if we, the parents, could be celebrated for our sleepless nights and snot smeared shirts as well as for giving a great presentation or doing something fantastic in the office. However, the reality is, as many working mums know, very different. The boss and clients don't want to know about your breakthrough with the potty training or junior's results in the exams. While your blog might contain seemingly innocuous recollections of nappy days, they might not help with your place in the workplace pecking order.

Equally, if the reality of most of your life is far too Clark Kent for you to blog about, then going online can give you the chance to be Superman for a while without the necessity to put your pants on top of your trousers. That's it – you can start any number of blogs on any subject you fancy. How liberating is that? You might hang up your work uniform and reveal your buzzing secret life as a sex-toy reviewer, you could talk about your radical proposals for world domination through poetry or, even, bring something new to the debate on organic food.

One of the most famous undercover bloggers – Belle de Jour – revealed her secret life and told the world how her Lois Lane took off her knickers altogether. Her adventures as a high-class call girl in London became so well known they were published in two volumes of memoirs and turned into a TV series starring Billie Piper. Speculation about the real Belle was ferocious. For a long time no one – not even her literary agent – knew her real identity.

Belle was the pseudonym of research scientist Dr Brooke Magnanti who works in the specialist areas of developmental neurotoxicology and cancer epidemiology. After years of speculation her identity was on the brink of being exposed so she had no choice but to 'out' herself in an interview in *The Times*.

Keeping the lid on the real her for such a long time took a huge amount of effort and subterfuge. She made sure there was no 'paper trail' or whiff of who she really was. Speaking to India Knight in *The Times* she said: 'Also, I started writing in 2003; I was one of the first bloggers to be anonymous. People weren't used to it. It was relatively easy for us to get our resources together and keep me anonymous. By the time other anonymous bloggers came along, people were looking out for them — they were under a lot more scrutiny.'

So, these days, maintaining a secret persona – even if it doesn't hit the dizzy heights of Brooke's – requires a degree of planning. Be careful to use separate email accounts and log-ins, keep your Twitter accounts apart and watch what clues you give away. Absolute secrecy requires great control.

Over in an entirely different corner of the blogosphere to Ms de Jour, Bumbling has found that as her blog became more successful, it was increasingly difficult to keep it quiet. Her blog has now been nominated for awards and she's been invited to speak at conferences. Secrecy is vanishing. 'I wasn't outed, but I did have to confess in general terms to a number of people, including my ex-husband,' she said. 'It became too difficult to explain where review products were coming from, or why I was attending [bloggers' conference] Cybermummy! But I've given the address to very few people.

'I'm getting less anonymous. I still won't use my name or Moo's on the blog or Twitter. But people within the [blogging] community know me, and I'm starting to let people I know in real life know about the online me.'

So far, we've talked about one's individual privacy. To a greater extent you can do what you like with your own secrets – but other peoples are a different matter.

What's the position when you blog about, say, your children or colleagues who don't have a say in the matter. My own rule is that I don't put my kids 'out there' for the world to find. That is, I do use their photos but not their names and as their surnames aren't the same as mine they won't be found on a search engine. Their online privacy will be up to them to squander when they're old enough, until then, it's my responsibility.

As far as other grown-ups are concerned, I try to only tell my own story, not other people's. There are several reasons for this. Firstly, it's not fair – if they want to humiliate themselves, confess or clamber out of the closet, that's their business not mine. Secondly, unless I'm going to offer someone a right of reply I have no right to make a claim about them. Perhaps this is an old-fashioned journalistic idea, but when I trained, if you said something about someone you had to tell them what you were doing and give them the opportunity to defend themselves or explain. It may be going out of fashion, but I believe it makes for balanced reporting – and blogging.

Now listen, I want to tell you a secret.

It's hard not to be drawn to a whisper, a rumour or the notion that there's something new and fresh being unwrapped for the first time. But the minute secrets are published on the internet they have taken their first baby steps to not being secrets any longer. So, share your secrets – as long as you're sure they are yours to share – it'll feel fantastic for a while, but just be aware that some secrets have a habit of coming back and biting you on the bottom.

Legal issues (copyright, libel)
You might be tempted to flick past this chapter with an air of 'I'm only fiddling about on my blog, why should I worry about the law?' about you. But it doesn't matter how humble and domestic your wee blog is, you're still publishing it and publishing – rather than scribbling something and putting it in a drawer – means that you have to follow the rules too.

But before you give the whole thing up as too complicated and scary, don't worry. In the words of various codes of practice, keep things 'legal, decent, honest and truthful'.

Actually I'm not going to worry too much about decent here. I suggest that if you're going to break decency regulations in your blogs, this is possibly not the book for you. However, if there's going to be swearing or discussions of an, ahem, adult nature on your blog, it's probably a good idea to warn those of a nervous disposition before they start reading.

Let's start with one of the most basic blog rules – don't steal. It might not actually feel like theft, but if you use someone else's words or photos without asking that's exactly what it is. You could always ask them and, in many cases, they'll say yes. Otherwise, come up with your own, after all, that's part of the point of the exercise, isn't it?

I'm all for people who have blogs to have opinions, lively opinions at that. However, they must be your opinions and what you believe about something must be the truth. If it isn't then you could be committing libel which is a crime. Libel is when you make a claim about something or someone that is not true and puts them in a negative light. It may even be something you believe, but if it isn't true and damages the reputation of someone – or their business – then it is still libel. If you're not sure about the truth, then find out the facts. There isn't really any protection in passing on information you learned on someone else's blog.

Equally you are responsible for the legality or otherwise of the comments made on your blog. You're still the publisher, even if the comment clearly comes from someone else.

Pay attention to the rules. When you sign up with any organization (your blog host platform, Twitter and so on), you agree to their terms and conditions. I know none of us actually stops to read all the text before ticking the box, but there are occasions when it's worth checking. For example, Facebook currently doesn't like you using their functionality to enter a giveaway competition. That means they don't want you saying 'like my page on Facebook to be in with a chance to win something marvelous'.

That brings me to competitions. The minute someone has to part with money to enter your competition, it becomes gambling and a veritable tsunami of regulations will be unleashed on you. Best to make any contests on your blog free-to-enter giveaways and games of skill.

Having said that, there may be occasions where organisations – often large ones with legal departments – may try to intimidate you into taking down a post or retracting what you've said. Don't let them. You are entitled to have your say and just because they don't like it, doesn't make it libel.

The other place you need to make sure your blog activities are above board is with the tax person. If you earn from your blog, it's income and must be declared. You could be liable to pay tax or it may affect the benefits you can claim. It is worth remembering that you can claim your costs, computer, subscriptions and so on against this.

Blogging dos and don'ts
Do pause for a moment and consider who will read your blog. Exposing your very soul to the pages of your diary every night is one thing, but whilst doing it on the web might seem similar, it can be a very different experience. Imagine everyone you know reading your most intimate thoughts: your boss, your mother-in-

law, your lover or your children. That gives you a bit of a shivery feeling, doesn't it?

Perhaps from the privacy of your own sofa/desk/smart phone, you think noone is really watching or, even, that noone cares, but it's worth remembering that, however dull you think your pontification is, anyone could read it.

Never blog about work unless you know what you are doing. While blogging can be a marvelous escape from the nine-to-fivery, it's worth considering the effect of what you write on your employer and your colleagues. A new word has sneaked into our language – dooced – after the famous blogger who fell foul of her employer. Borrow her learning curve, please.

Heather B. Armstrong was a Los Angeles-based web designer who started a blog called *Dooce* in 2001. Her openness and foul-mouthed, but funny, turn of phrase, quickly got her a raft of followers. For a while she talked cheerfully about her colleagues and her Mormon family. None of it was flattering.

First her brother googled her name and found what she'd said about the tribe. Her family didn't talk to her for months; now she'll only say things about her family that she'd say to their faces.

A few months later, her boss got an anonymous tip-off about Dooce.com – so named, by the way, for her inability to spell 'dude' – and wasted no time in giving Heather the push. And dooced entered the urban dictionary to describe anyone who has been sacked for what they wrote on their blog.

Heather counselled: 'My advice to you is BE YE NOT SO STUPID. Never write about work on the internet unless your boss knows and sanctions the fact that YOU ARE WRITING ABOUT WORK ON THE INTERNET.'

Dooce.com is still going strong with apparently some 300,000 readers every day. The blog now supports Heather and her husband. It's unlikely, though, that latter-day doocing will yield such a happy ending.

Heather's words are wise. I like to think I use the tell-it-to-their face filter. Before each post, I pause and ask myself 'if I wasn't such a cowardy custard, would I like to say these exact words to the subject of my post?' If the answer is yes, then I press the 'publish' button, if not then delete.

Do not reveal more than you are comfortable with. The other question to ask before clicking that tempting little button is: 'Do I care that anyone knows what I'm about to reveal about myself?' Again, if you have reservations then don't publish.

I know I'm all for glasnost and getting all out there in the open, but sometimes the affect can take you by surprise. For example, what if your kid's headteacher learns about your teenage sexual habits, your mum finds out what drugs you took and that person who has just been recommending you for a work project discovers that you are a secret slattern? And all of that is before you get into the well-known quicksand of religion, politics and what your child-rearing philosophy is.

For example, I'm quite happy to let the world know that I've had a miscarriage, a failed marriage and post-natal depression, but some of my acquaintances, I have learned, don't want to know that. Following a revelation, mundane encounters have seemed, to my perhaps paranoid eyes, to have taken on another dimension. It's like they are actually saying 'here's a package you have to sign for', but thinking 'this woman is a real fruitcake and I know what she did when she was 20'.

My nuts-and-bolts practical brain knows that it's not my problem and it doesn't make any difference whatsoever to my life, so if they don't like it, they can just shove off and read someone else's post. But it's an unsettling feeling. A former colleague once said he thought I ought to stop writing personal things in my blog because it made him uncomfortable. I suggested that, instead, he should stop reading. He did, but our relationship has never been quite the same since.

My husband, a deceptively sensitive and perceptive man, once said: 'The reason some men go weird around pregnant women is that the bump is proof that they had sex and they can't think past that.' He may be right, but if 'some men' want to get their knickers in a twist about what I've written, I really don't care.

The bottom line is that it's important to know what your own rules are. Do you mention your children, your mental health, your job, your family, your sex life? And if so what effect is it going to have not just on your nearest and dearest, but everyone you know?

At risk of sounding like been-there-done-that Old Mother Time, I'd also like to point out that what might seem very like a very heated and significant thing this week will probably pass into nothingness with time. So try to pause and think about whether the trouble you are likely to cause yourself will be worth it in, say, a year. My 'rules' are as follows:

1. Do protect your children online. There is a degree of squeamishness about children on blogs. How much of them can you reveal? For most parents, the most immediate issue is clearly to keep them safe. Therefore, I don't use my sons' names and because their second names are different to mine, it isn't going to be easy to identify them. I turn up in search engines, but they don't.

I do use their photos because, to me, they are too lovely not to. It's also an excellent way of letting family and friends see what they've been up to. I have had a long think about this but I really don't believe they are in any kind of danger because of this. If someone was hell-bent on finding them with some sinister intent, then they'd be able to do that blog or no blog. After all, they're out of my sight at school, cubs, nursery and the childminder. They are no more vulnerable to a bogeyman than my siblings and I were a generation ago.

Perhaps greater concern might be for the kids themselves and what you write or publish of their lives. After all they didn't ask to have the cute picture of them paddling in the lavatory or dressed as Tigger on show for all the world. If you give them a cuddly pet name or reveal their teenage habits, how will they feel about that? Ultimately, how much of their lives is it fair to share?

My older boys both now know I write on the internet and occasionally ask to see the latest missive. Generally, they find it all rather dull. However, I don't hide anything from them and if there was something they didn't like I'd take it down. Imagine how a teenager will feel if his or her classmates discover that you keep an online family album. And I quite accept that I may have to change my view on this as they get older. If my blog were causing them anything more than a faint discomfort, I'd have to do something about it.

There are, however, true child protection issues in amongst the blushes and potential ribbing from classmates. In separated or otherwise fighting families, blogs can provide a rich seam of ammunition. I know it may be hard to consider such an outcome in the flush of an amusing or irreverent blog post idea, but a little ponder of the ramifications is wise.

2.   Do a blog safety check. You know when your tiny baby starts to get mobile and you have to do the safety audit of the house? Remember: can they reach the door, the DVD player, the cooker knobs or the expensive and fragile ornaments? Well a blog safety audit is recommended. Don't make your plans based on who you actually know read your blog either. You don't know who your silent readers are. Bear in mind that thinking 'it's OK such-and-such doesn't go online so I can say what I like' is very, very foolish.

And as with a crawling tot who develops into a climber and walker, the safety checks need to keep abreast of developments. You don't want to get caught out by a wobbly shelf. Just as you can hardly imagine your, at the moment, predictable slow moving baby climbing up a book case, out of a window or opening a really boring and complicated looking cupboard, you consider that it's just possible. Same thing online.

You might not think anyone will use your private trivia against you, but they could. Anyone you are in dispute with might be rubbing their hands together at your entertaining revelation of household mayhem. Your political, moral or social assertions could quite quickly be turned around to smack you in the face.

I'm really not saying don't post freely. That after all is the joy, just apply a caution before you press publish.

3. Do be sure you really want a fight. If, like me, an argument of any kind can leave you feeling bruised and battered, then that caution filter must also be at least considered if you're wading into a hair-trigger debate. You know the sort – abortion, independence, immigration and feminism feature highly. There are some topics that once you broach you will draw an inevitable and vitriolic response. The people who perhaps used to restrict themselves to writing ferociously letters to newspapers – often in green ink – now find similar sport responding to blog posts. Just be prepared with either your defence or your course of action. The strength of emotion expressed through the safety of the keyboard can be breath-taking, as can the frankness of response. On the other hand, if you're in the mood for a good scrap then you'll find plenty happy to give you a virtual square go.

4. Do keep yourself safe. The other consideration may be to keep yourself safe from crime. A cyber-savvy burglar might be very keen on photos of the inside of your house that show the door key on a string just through the letter box. Or they might be delighted to learn you leave your window open at night so the cat can come and go. Equally with your kids, it's a valid debate to consider the correct age for leaving a child home alone, but just don't tell the world you're going to do it Tuesday next week.

5. Don't forget who you really are. Don't get lost in the personality of your blog. What I mean by this is that if you are, for example, a mummy blogger then make sure you don't lose the person behind the parent persona. Terri Blodell warned, those who are exclusively 'mummy bloggers' need to beware that they

could be getting lost behind the title. They need to be sure they are complete people first and 'mummies' second.

Terri added: 'Mummies are human beings as well. We all do other things. It's very easy to get into that category and get stuck in it. Then when the kids are older and going off to do their own things and becoming more independent, that's when mummy starts to feel "what's there left for me?"

'It's important to maintain a balance. And that will teach your children about balance too. They need to be grateful and look for the positives in other people and in themselves.'

Balance can also be an issue if your blog becomes a ghetto of whinge. Anonymous blogger Bumbling of *Bumbling Along* started blogging when she was going through a difficult time in real life: 'Keeping it completely shielded from real life friends was useful, as I felt I could pour my heart out online (and I've had a tough year) but I also felt it ended up throwing me into a downward cycle. I didn't really like the online me at one point. If you're not in a good place, it can make you wallow, as there's no filter, no "what would people think of me if they read this".'

So she paused and restarted her blog – and one for her daughter – but with a slightly more public presence this time. It means she is more conscious of what she's committing to internet, which she considers a good thing.

6. Do tell the truth. Be sure that the you on your blog matches up with the one in the real world. At work, if you've bent the truth or omitted something possibly significant that you then blog about, don't be surprised if the consequences are messy or embarrassing. Imagine that, just to keep in we understand, you told your boss that you can't stand reality TV/Manchester United/binge drinking. You made out you're much more likely to be giving intelligent contribution to your local book group or visiting the art gallery. Then someone happens to come across your blog where you give lively and thorough analysis of Simon Cowell's latest offering/details of your horror hangover/praise of Alex Ferguson etc. It's not going to look good, is it?

7.   Don't steal. Beware posting things that don't belong to you. I don't just mean photos and words that you didn't create, that I mentioned earlier. I mean information you've learned that isn't actually yours to pass on, just because you know it.

Trade secrets would fall under this category. A juicy piece of industry information someone passed on in confidence would count. Blogging isn't the same as phoning your friend and saying: 'Guess what I heard?' It might feel cosy and familiar, but it isn't always.

Many of my friends work for national media and often share the most delicious bits of gossip and insider knowledge but it would be more than their jobs are worth for me to pass them on, tempting as it might be. I wouldn't break their trust.

8.   Don't tell other people's stories. Equally, other people's news is for them to broadcast not you. There's no law against it, but it's just, in my opinion, not fair to announce other people's sexuality, pregnancy, relationship status or employment news. Yes, we all like a good gossip, but – even if you think the subject deserves everything they get – you just shouldn't do it. In any case if what you post isn't true, you'll find there is a law against it.

The same rules apply for publishing on a blog as in other forms of media – things must be legal, decent, honest and fair. So if you make a claim, be sure it's true and that you can prove it if called upon.

And even if your observations meet all of the guidelines – and are your opinion alone – it's entirely possible that some individuals will be less than thrilled to find themselves with a starring role in your latest post.

9.   Do be clear who you're talking about. If you make it plain who you are talking about you will only offend one person, whereas if you are vague about who you're having a pop at, then there could be a cloud of confusion as several people think they are your target. How you handle that is your call, but it's worth

remembering that what you think is a crystal clear reference to a time and place in your head might mean something else to others.

Keith Kendrick who blogs at *The Reluctant Housedad* learned an important lesson in the early days of his blog – and his new role as stay-at-home dad. He had been bewildered by his seeming status as persona non grata at the school gates. The other parents – mostly mums – didn't seem to want to invite him into their gang. Eventually, when asked, he explained how his wife was now the breadwinner. There were sighs of relief as the mums had speculated all manner of mishap and domestic strife. He was welcomed into the fold until he blogged about the exchange.

A little later one of the mums sent a 'warning shot across his bows' that she, and the others, were watching him and his blog. Keith said: 'I think when you start doing a blog you think you're the only person in the world who will read it. You don't research your potential audience or the fact that so many communities exist – communities that are very tight and loyal to one another.

'In my case, I thought it would showcase my writing (I am a former magazine editor and wanted to make a living as a freelance writer). But you learn pretty quickly what the rules are. The material you write about attracts a similar audience of like-minded bloggers. It is statistical suicide to offend them because word spreads quickly and you lose the very people who can help you market – through Twitter, word-of-mouth etc – your musings.

'You can only write about what you know i.e. what's closest to home, but if the things you know are the things that are potentially offensive to those closest to home, then they will find out. I have discovered – just in passing – that my tweets are followed by some of my family, my friends, my neighbours, parents from my children's schools and even people in the pub where I drink. They never "announced" they were following me – they just mentioned it in passing. It's like a heads-up: be careful what you write, make sure it doesn't offend us, and make sure it's true. Because if it isn't, we'll be down on you like a ton of bricks!'

10. Do be aware that with blogging, as with all good things, you can get too much of it. Especially in the first flush of your love-affair with blogging and internet communities, it's possible to think it's the only thing that really matters, that your sparkly new internet friends are much, much more important than the feet-of-clay, flesh-and-blood ones. And it's true you can think that your fellow bloggers are the only people who properly 'get' you, laugh at your jokes and realise what a clever, talented person you are. Of course they do. All they have to do is give a pleasing and flattering one or two-line response to your latest outpouring. It will have taken them a minute at most and you will be quite disproportionately flattered. Beware, this is very seductive. Your significant other, your children and your pets will quite quickly become very disenchanted with your online success when it means they only ever see you in profile by the glow of your laptop screen. Please don't forget that they should be the people who come first, so don't get obsessed. In some rare cases an infatuation has become an obsession that needs proper treatment, but not often. Clinical psychotherapist Terri Bodell said: 'People can become obsessed by blogging and the internet, but, then again, if they're going to get obsessed by an online community, they're going to have an obsessive personality in the first place.

'People can get too obsessed by these things when they lose track of "proper" people outside the internet – they forget to talk to those at home.'

There are dangers of getting in with the wrong people: of falling for someone who isn't as they seem. Taking the usual care about revealing too much in a blog, the dangers are no greater now than they ever were. Meeting people for the first time always required a degree of faith in human nature and your own judgement.

'You need to trust your instincts and listen to your gut, the same as in real life. If you do that, then being online is a brilliant way of contacting other people particularly those in the same situation. You can help them and they can help you. Just go with your gut and don't doubt yourself,' added Terri.

Using Twitter
When there is dialogue, you have a degree of power.' Sarah Brown

Sarah Brown, wife of former prime minister Gordon Brown, is something of a superstar on Twitter. She has more than a million followers and has used Twitter to great effect both during her husband's time of office and after. Speaking at Cybermummy – a conference for parent bloggers – she explained why Twitter was her social media of choice despite having already written blog posts on the Number Ten website. Sarah said she considered taking up blogging or using Facebook but rejected them because they didn't suit the style of on-the-go snappy communication she was after: 'I wanted to support Gordon, but I didn't want to go through people. And I thought 140 characters was within my concentration span.

'Through Twitter I could shine a light on our day-to-day life. I could be myself and I could identify my own voice.'

Twitter is a social media phenomena where it is possible to send a short message that will be read by the people who follow you or the people who are searching for what's in your message. Imagine everyone you've met in the last two years is updating their Facebook statuses so fast the new messages are flowing like a river. If you spot something that interests you, it's possible to do the Twitter equivalent of saying 'oi, tell me more'. But generally it babbles away waiting for you to dip your toe in to find out who is tweeting what.

What's Twitter to you? Is it a sea of irrelevant chatter or a life-line, like having a pocketful of friends?

The broadsheets describe Twitter as the 'micro-blogging site'. You don't have a site of your own. You have a profile and a place you can tweet. You also have a place to see everything that anyone you follow has tweeted lately.

Twitter isn't really a blog, but it does share many characteristics and often goes hand in hand. Your Twitter account can reveal exactly the slice of you that you choose to reveal, just the same as a 'proper' blog. It can be found by anyone and, while there isn't an archive as such, your recent tweets are there for all the world to see.

The real advantage of Twitter is twofold – its immediacy and its searchability. You can have instant feedback, perhaps offering sympathy or support, or just the sense there is someone else on the planet who gives a hoot, even though you know they don't actually know your real name, what your face looks like or where you live. For example, the day I wrote this I was going to a Take That concert, purely for work you understand. I wasn't sure about how to get there or where to park, but within minutes Twitter people had given me a solution. I've also just had a lively and entertaining conversation with someone who is tweeting as if they were a talking dog.

I have the vision of us all beavering away on our own – working from home, looking after kids, sitting on trains or even in the office – and Twitter gives us a little human contact without any of the hassle. Someone to laugh at your joke without having to get involved in awkward water cooler etiquette. There's no obligation and you don't have to deal with that 'oh hell, I know you from somewhere, but I just can't remember where or what your name is' moment the next time.

Tweeters are always there with an instant opinion or some advice. They mean someone sensible is always on hand to say whether the blue or the red is best, staying or going, or cheese or chicken. And the real beauty is you can ignore it without upsetting anyone. It's the freedom of talking to strangers but reduced to a snappy 140 characters.

But Twitter isn't always as superficial as that – there is far more to it than who is having what for lunch and the magnitude of the contents of junior's latest nappy. (Don't you know as a parent who blogs, you have a contractual obligation to mention baby poo at least once a month?)

There are some real warm proper friendships blooming on Twitter. Just take a look at what's going on there any evening. You can see that people are simply settling down on their sofas with their internet-connecting doodah of choice and a large glass of something to tweet their mates. How good is that? It provides a lifeline of friendship to those who, for whatever reason, just don't have that.

It has all the benefit of popping in to a local pub or coffee shop without any of the need for a baby sitter, negotiations with your other half, awkward moments when there's no one you want to talk to or need, even, to get dressed. What's especially tempting is that you can pick the conversations to butt into or just start your own.

Sometimes Twitter provides something that feels like a companion settling down on the sofa next to you ready to provide amusing analysis of the latest reality television show. How could they possible want to vote HIM off and why did she ever think that dress would look good?

I'd go so far as to say that Twitter is the best thing that can happen to a temporarily lonely person. In the words of that old hippy Max Ehrmann's *Desiderata of Happiness*:

'Do not distress yourself with dark imaginings.
Many fears are born of fatigue and loneliness.'

True as it is, it's easier for him to say than it is to do something about. Solitude, whether from circumstance, choice or any kind of mental funk, isn't very easy to escape.

Single parents are stuck at home unable to find babysitters, the recession means social outings are often first for the chop and various circumstances see folk stranded in far flung places away from nearest and dearest. It's made worse by the fact that social muscles very quickly wither and become feeble. It doesn't take long before the idea of entering a room full of people just talking to each other and joining in is utterly terrifying.

And blogging – wonderful as it is – is by its nature a solitary activity. It's so much easier to sit at home and type your ideas onto the eagerly attentive keyboard, than it is to tell them to real people. Real people might not like them, they might not like you, they might even find them dull which may actually be worse. Obviously these thoughts are the kind of dark imaginings Mr. E. was talking about, but they are troublesome nonetheless.

Here's where Twitter comes in. Think of it as the games hall of sociability, the gym of interaction and the playing field of people skills. It's a safe, non-scary place to practice talking to people again about something other than whether or not you need help packing your shopping into bags. You can sit on the sidelines and observe if you feel like it and no one will even notice you're there. In the real world, they're probably not going to notice you either but it never feels that way.

You could initiate a conversation without that awful sickening sweep of shame you feel when no one picks it up, or you stutter, or choose just that moment to dribble your tea down your front. On Twitter if no one replies, the chances are they didn't read what you said or it wasn't their thing – just a matter of fact rather than a faux pas. Try again, or re-phrase and have another go. And they have no idea you stammered and slurped.

Hello @interestingperson is a much less intimidating way of getting into a lively conversation than standing on the fringe of a group and saying 'excuse me'. And then before you know it you're chatting away as if you were good at it. There's no blushing, hesitating or awkward moments when you're so overcome by the fact people are listening that you forget where you're going with your sentence.

Gordon Darroch who blogs at *Unreal Domain*, *Autistic Dad* and *Words for Press* said: 'Twitter is a hugely effective forum and I've used it a lot, especially for the journalism blog. Getting retweeted by people with lots of followers is like super-strength fertiliser for a blog. But you need to tweet carefully: people on

Twitter have their spam radar on high alert. I have a basic rule of three plugs and you're out, otherwise you quickly start to annoy people.'

Here are a few of the things I've learned about Twitter:

1. It's not the same as Facebook.
Here's where a lot of people stumble. We've all been doing Facebook for so long, our kids are on it, our parents. We know how it works – update your status (using the 'Jane Bloggs is...' construction), share your photos and 'like' things. We understand that people will typically check their Facebook friends' status at least once a day to catch up on the news. We know people 'like' things because they want to be in with the in crowd or they want to keep up with the gossip, or, perhaps, they really genuinely like things. There's no desperate immediacy about it. We also know that – once sufficient attention has been paid to the rules and check boxes – it's possible to control who sees what. Photos loaded to Facebook skulk around there until someone does something to remove them.

2. Twitter is a fast-flowing stream
Once you follow more than about a dozen people who tweet regularly, it's impossible to keep track of everything they say. Indeed, I'd go as far as to suggest that way lies madness. You may as well drop your children off at the social services department and the dog at the kennels now, because you won't have time to look after them. The world – or at least mine – is cluttered up enough without adding too much pointless observation and opinion from people I don't even know. (Although some observation and opinion will prove entertaining and informative, it's just that I must choose when I see it and how much.) I find it helpful to think of it as a river, where you can dip in your toe when it suits. The advantage of this is it is sort of self cleaning. If you say something daft or get into an unseemly scrap, while the evidence won't vanish, it will be swept so far downstream that only stalkers and journalists will bother tracking it down.

Blogging for happiness

3.   FF, RT and other mysterious things

Twitter has already got its own language, largely because with only 140 characters to tell your story you don't want to waste them on spelling out 'Friday Follow' or 'Retweet'. So a shorthand of sorts has appeared. It's not like the nasty text language that infected things for a while. Someone is unlikely to say 'C U 2moro m8', although you may find a little LOLing or even the occasional LMAO.

4.   Terms you will need to know

Follow   If you follow someone you can see everything they say in your Twitter stream.

Name   Your Twitter name (mine is @Ellen27) is what people use to call you. It's a snappy version of your address and postcard. You can change it if you want, but that could cause confusion.

RT   A retweet. That is to send someone else's tweet on so your followers can see it. It's a shorthand way of saying 'look at this, it's interesting', or simply showing your support.

FF   Follow Friday. What? Yes. It's a Twitter thing. You suggest to the people who follow you who else they should be following. Along the lines of 'meet Amanda, she's brilliant, you'll really like her'.

DM   Direct mail. If you follow someone and they follow you back, you can send them a direct message that no one else can see.

A hashtag. By putting a hashtag – or # – in a tweet before a phrase, it makes it easier to track all the tweets on that subject. For example it could be #superbowl #royalwedding or #xfactor. It might seem a bit daft, but it does make life easier if you're trying to follow some breaking news or, even, the thrilling final of a reality TV talent show. Event organisers often pick a hashtag for all relevant tweets.

How to blog

Other terms include 'tweeps', which is the term for a collection of people who tweet; 'fail whale', which is what you get on your screen when Twitter stops working (which it does from time to time, usually just when you'd really, really like it to work); and 'trends/trending', which is a list of what most people are talking about on Twitter right now this minute. You'll see it just there on the right. It changes quite quickly, often to what's happening in the world. Twitter followers are the first to discover who has died, who is tipped for which team and which celeb has done what with whom. In the future, your 'what were you doing when Diana/JFK died moment?' will almost certainly be 'checking Twitter'.

5.   There are rules
Manners are maketh a tweep apparently. For example, if someone suggests you as a FF (Friday Follow) person, it's good form to thank them. Likewise if someone retweets your message or otherwise does you a service. 'Pleases' make things easier too. While butting in is hunky-dory, it's nice to excuse yourself as you do so. If you don't like someone, you have the option of just not following them any longer.

And there is the law. Theoretically, Twitter is subject to the same rules as more traditional publishing – at the time of writing it hasn't been properly tested, but it is worth considering before you spread or pass on sensational information.

6.   It's funny
One of the things that lifts Twitter out of the confusion of the modern and relentless is that it's very funny. At any point there may be a hashtag topic trending with one-line laughs. For example, today #scottishfilms is doing the rounds with such gems as 'Ross County For Old Men' and 'Buckfast at Tiffany's'.

7.   If there's a party you don't need an invite
A Twitter party isn't something that happens in an aviary when there's an extra portion of birdseed. It's a gathering on Twitter at

an arranged time to discuss an arranged subject. More fun than it sounds.

8.   And Phil Collins was right.
He sang *Follow Me, Follow You* long before Twitter was even an impulse on a circuit board (do you get impulses on circuit boards? See, I told you I wasn't technical). But he was right in terms of Twitter. Following someone isn't vital, but it is friendly – like taking your turn at the bar or returning the invite for dinner.

This is all very well but what's it got to do with blogs? Well, if the internet is the landscape and blogs the trees, then Twitter could be the forest plants growing in between. Maybe. Implausible and unwieldy metaphors aside, most bloggers use Twitter. They talk to each other on Twitter and use it to let the world know what they've just blogged about. I follow a few of my favourite bloggers just so I know when they've said something new.

I also talk to tweeps to help me gather my thoughts – and theirs – on whatever topic I'm about to write.

Conversely, I've found some great blogs by having a closer look at someone I was talking to. Bloggers tend to have their blog address on their profile. It follows that if you like the cut of someone's jib in 140 characters then you'll probably enjoy what they have to say when they have more room.

I know Twitter is the brash upstart of the internet and it isn't for everyone, but I couldn't be without it.

Making time to blog
The double dangers are that you let blogging take over your life – believe me, it's addictive – or that you are a bit inconsistent in your approach. My advice to stop these dangers from happening is quite simple: set a realistic timetable for your own blog activity.

As well as providing structure to your blogging week, which will also help your readers, it can help keep your blog from taking over your life. From the position of considering 'to blog, or not to blog', it might seem inconceivable that this little quirky online hobby can become so all consuming, yet it can. Once readers come, and they will, many bloggers feel a self-imposed pressure to keep delivering regular posts. The more feedback they get, the better it feels and so they keep going. 'For my readers,' they say like there are hoards of them just logging on in the morning ready for your next offering. Well, perhaps that's an exaggeration, but a blog really ought to be blogged in regularly and when it isn't a blogger is inclined to get antsy.

Nadine Hill, time management expert, blogger and author of *I Don't Have Time To Write*, has come to the rescue with the notion of a blog timetable to take hold of the thing again and provide structure: 'In our time-pressed, busy lives setting a blog timetable is crucial to maintain some control over your blog output whilst keeping the blog in its place – as an enhancer of your life rather than a pressure that is trying to take over it.

'The structure of setting days and committing this to paper allows you space to gather your thoughts so you have time to construct quality posts and also makes it easier to see the type of posts you are putting out in sequence. This is important so you can vary the type of posts being published (vlogs, review posts, photo stories etc). In this case, putting some structure around your blog actually has the effect of setting you free.'

Nadine suggests deciding how frequently you are planning to update your blog – in my case three times a week plus a bonus photo at the weekend. Then she recommends having a look at the kinds of content to ensure there's a healthy mix, if that's what you're after. And, finally, the key to the success of the thing is to get your posts ready ahead of time, that way you can relax – you're organised for the next few posts.

The last time I spoke to Nadine, she told me she had the next month's blog posts all prepared and ready to go. That's organisation to a level I could only imagine, but it does mean she can enjoy her forthcoming holiday without letting her blog get in the way.

It doesn't work for everyone. My blog posts are invariably more of a reaction to something or other and, consequently, subject to change. However, I have adopted some of Nadine's recommendations and usually have a couple of posts 'in the bag' for the times when life gets in the way of blogging.

However, there aren't any rules. Your blog can take up as much of your time and head space as you want it to. Remember that it's your blog and you're the boss. It might well be the one part of your life where you feel truly yourself, confident and in control.

Blogging for money

'I am fiercely loyal to those willing to put their money where my mouth is.'
Paul Harvey

Let's get this out of the way first. Anyone who likes to write harbours a fantasy about being spotted by a publisher and turned into the next big thing. Our version of Harry Potter or Bridget Jones is just waiting to be launched on a thunderstruck world, of course. But the point is; it's fantasy. It's the literary equivalent of a tall dark handsome stranger finding a lonely woman in the supermarket cleaning products aisle and declaring she's the one he wants to share his immense fortune with. As they say, it ain't gonna happen, not in this lifetime.

Yes, yes. I know it has happened to some people. Their blogs were 'found', their books published and now they're doing quite nicely, but it really isn't the norm.

Some bloggers are squeamish about any form of commercialisation on their precious blogs. They are uncomfortable that their free-wheeling creation should be sullied by big (or small) business. That's just fine, but, if that's you, you won't find much of interest in this section so you best just move along now.

Have they gone now? Good.

So, the reality is that it's unlikely that a blog will allow you to give up your day job. Unless, of course, that and nothing else is what you are setting out to accomplish with your blog. What it might do – aside from earning an extra few pounds – is help you get a better day job, or help your day job improve.

Carol Smith, who blogs at *Parent Panel*, *New Mummy's Tips* and *Dance Without Sleeping*, is something of an expert at making blogging pay: 'I make money from my blogs in several ways – direct ads, ads from *Glam Media* that work on page views (the number of times someone clicks through an advert to the place being advertised), sponsored posts for companies that contact me directly, sponsored posts for eBuzz and paid text links in the side bar.

'I have a page on my blogs that informs PRs etc that I take on ads and sponsored posts. They tend to come to me. I haven't really had to promote too much to get them. Though I am pimping my new blog at the moment.

'I have been blogging for several years and I have built up a good reputation, plus I have decent traffic which helps. If you really want to make money from blogging it is achievable but its hard work.'

The following sections will look at ways you can follow Carol's example and give your bank balance (or career) a boost by means of your blog.

Advertising

Let's start with the ways you can make a quid or two – or 'monetizing your blog' as current speak goes. The most obvious, I suppose, is advertising. And the most direct way of doing this is to make a deal with a company who give you hard cash in exchange for being featured on your blog. Many bloggers do very well with this approach although it's far too businessy for some of us.

The medium may be new but the principal isn't: if you can offer a business something special with access to your followers then you can charge a reasonable price for it. For example, if you are an expert fisherman and blog regularly about innovations in waders or fishhooks and have an engaged population of anglers hanging on your every word, then you could quite reasonably expect to reel in (yes, I did) a fishing rod manufacturer.

To a certain extent the potential of your blog to make advertising revenue depends on what the people who read it have in common and, more importantly, if they coincide with the target clientele of a business that wants to advertise.

So a good natured, general blog about all aspects of your life may not be the best vehicle for raising advertising money unless the commercial target is readers of good natured blogs about life. I fear it rarely will be. In order to make real money from a blog, you need a niche that is specific and ripe for commercial exploitation.

Entrepreneurial Erica Douglas is a blogger who has turned her blog, *littlemummy.com*, into the start of a lucrative business. She said: 'I think anyone is capable of making money from a blog but you need to choose a good niche, build a loyal audience and know how to market it all.'

To Erica thinking commercially comes easily, but I'm not a natural business person and the idea of cold-calling a company and saying 'erm, I've got a blog please give me money' makes me feel quite queasy. Not, the notion of advertising though, just the process of getting it. Luckily there are organisations that are more than happy to help.

Blogger Krista Madden launched *Handpicked Media* when she was frustrated by her inability to find a network for niche websites and blogs in the UK. She had struggled to discover the right agency to represent her site *beautyandthedirt.com* so, eventually, created her own.

Now the *Handpicked Community* is a network of blogs loosely under the theme of fashion, beauty, culture, food, grooming and home. She and her team sell advertising that the bloggers can opt to carry, or not, depending on their sensibilities. Bloggers get 65 per cent of the revenue, which is generally measured by the number of people who click through the advert to the advertiser's site.

There are other sites doing similar. *Glam Media* negotiates with brands on behalf of their network members, but they require a fairly high minimum number of monthly visits to your blog before you can qualify. eBuzz is another organisation that lets brands pay to have their adverts or content on blogs across Europe.

The advantage of these agencies is that they do the selling, they establish the relationship with the brands and they run the show. All you can do is say yes or no to what they are offering and allow your blog to become an internet billboard. So, on the one hand it's easy, but on the other you are unlikely to be putting down the deposit on a yacht any time soon.

In a similar vein – that is easy advertising income – Google's AdSense is a common route to go down. Once you sign up adverts, in a format you dictate, are automatically delivered to your blog depending on the content therein. You earn tiny amounts with each click through to the advertiser. So, clearly, to be quids in you need to have lots of visitors moved by the adverts.

In summary, advertising works very well for some bloggers. However in order to sell space, you need to focus on the benefit to the advertiser. A little restraint is called for in placing ads on your blog, too many and your readers will stop coming to visit.

If you don't fancy the hard sell yourself, then use an agency, or even a computer programme, but you won't make so much money. And do bear in mind that bloggers often forget to remove adverts after the contracted period is over – by doing that your advertiser is getting something for nothing. Just saying.

Advertorials

From time to time, I take money to write a post, or rather I get paid to blog on a specific topic, or I earn money from writing about what someone else wants me to. Whatever way you phrase it, it sounds a bit sleazy, doesn't it?

Actually it's not really. Or I don't think so, after all I've been taking money for writing things – one way or another – for 20 years. But it's been going on for much, much longer than I've been using words to pay my bills. In newspapers or magazines they tend to be called advertorials or promotions. I can still remember my first one when I was a cub reporter on a paper called the *Rutherglen Reformer* back before there was even email – yes, I am that old. I had to write about how marvelous a local takeaway was. As the takeaway wasn't that handy I was faced with a choice: hang around the office until suppertime and trek out of my way to sample the funky foreign fare (I don't know why you have to alliterate in advertorials, but you just do) or get them to tell me what they sell and then use my imagination.

So there I was writing about my taste buds tingling as I sampled a spice sensation at the terrific takeaway and I had an epiphany... when you read something like this, it might not be true. What's that? I hear sharp intakes of breath. Look, the fabulous fast-food shop were paying for these words to be written, so, even if I sampled a colourful curry and found it was, in fact, dire not delightful, I was hardly going to say so.

Advertorial, like my tasty tale of the perfect pakora parlour, is clearly marked as such and paid for by the business. It is much the same as the blurb on a flyer or the menu. The only difference is that, written by journalists, it is, theoretically, a better class of adjective strewn prose.

As with print media, a blog should make it abundantly clear that a post has been paid for. You don't have to say how much, just that it has. I know that it might now seem that your opinion has been bought as well as the space on your blog, but, I'm afraid that's just the way it is. You might boast that the opinions on your blog are your own, but, deep, deep inside you know that's not true if you're paid to have them. If you don't want your pristine blog sullied by the smear of commerce, then don't take the money. That said, I believe most readers know and trust the voices on the blogs they follow and are happy to read – or ignore – a sponsored post so long as you are straight about it.

Blogging – commercially and just for fun – is only part of what I do. I write and I have to make some money at it. I trust the people who come to my blog would understand that.

How do you find these companies begging you to 're-view' their product? Good question. Having been loitering around the internet for a while, some come to me and ask. These days I only accept if it's something I'm genuinely interested in or, perhaps, would consider paying cash for.

Approaches can come direct from companies or through their PR and marketing agents. It is worth considering putting details of your terms, rates and policy on your blog in order that it's absolutely clear where you stand on these things. It does look more professional and can save time on approaches that clearly aren't suitable. Organisations such as *Handpicked Media*, *Glam* and *EBuzzing* all broker advertorial deals between business and bloggers.

My policy is that I'm happy to take advertorials, but I will clearly mark them as such. I also try to make sure they are written in a reasonably engaging way. Then I follow up with a 'real' post reasonably quickly afterwards so that the first post someone sees arriving at my blog, isn't a paid-for piece of puffery.

And a last word on disclosing when you're paid to write and when you're not. It's not just me saying this, it's the Office of Fair Trading. In December they ruled that bloggers must make it clear if a post was as a result of a commercial transaction. Heather Clayton, Senior Director of OFT's Consumer Group, said: 'The internet plays a key role in how people purchase products and services and the importance of online advertising continues to grow. The integrity of information published online is crucial so that people can make informed decisions on how to spend their money.

'We expect online advertising and marketing campaigns to be transparent so consumers can clearly tell when blogs, posts and microblogs have been published in return for payment or payment in kind. We expect this to include promotions for products and services as well as editorial content.'

Affiliates and working with brands
Affiliate marketing is one of those things that is not instantly possible to grasp. For me anyway, but perhaps I'm just a bit

dense about this. Actually it is a simple and very effective way of earning a little from your blog.

It describes a relationship where you promote someone's business on your blog and if one of your readers comes along and buys something from your affiliate partner, you get a cut. Imagine your friend has opened a sausage emporium. Another friend is pondering about what to feed the family. You suggest a pork sensation from your banger-making chum. When the second friend spends loads of money with your first friend, the first friend gives you something in return. Simple!

How do you set this up then? Well it could be directly with a company. For example, I have a bit of a thing about shoes that are fun and comfortable. Some would say I dress my toes like those of an overgrown toddler, but I don't care. Any fool, as my dad used to say, can be uncomfortable. And I'll always pick bright and shiny over boring, regardless of the context.

So I was particularly excited when Hotter, one of my favourite comfortable, yet colourful, shoes came to Glasgow. I contacted the company and told them so. They invited me to visit the shop and 'review' a pair of shoes. Which I did in glowing terms and stated clearly I'd been given a pair.

Later they suggested I might be interested in their affiliate scheme. Oh, yes. I agreed then rushed to Google to find out how it worked.

Through a third party business Affiliate Window, I can join a scheme that records everyone who clicks from my site to the comfy shoe shop to buy a pair and I will be rewarded each time.

There are agencies such as Click Bank, eJunkie or Affiliate Futures that make this happen in a very un-fussy way. Once again the key to this is finding things your readers will want to buy so having a niche makes this much easier.

Amazon was one of the first companies to get really good at affiliate marketing and they hold a patent for one of the clever e-shop widgets.

Of course, setting up shop for someone else isn't the only way of working with brands. Many bloggers become brand ambassadors. These are bloggers who establish a 'special', but usually commercial to some extent, relationship with a business. It may be that an organisation is sponsoring them, possibly to attend an event. Perhaps there's an agreement to support an initiative or charity.

This area between an advert and unbiased editorial is fairly grey, but in a good way. I don't see any problem with bloggers and business getting into bed together so long as everyone – readers included – understands what's going on.

As with any satisfactory relationship though, there will be a considerable amount of eyeing up and flirting going on first. It's as important to the brand that the bloggers they work with reflect what they are trying to do and are talking to, for them, the right kinds of people. Equally, a relationship with a product that means nothing to your hard-earned loyal readers will mean they'll ignore it and, at worst, stop visiting you, thinking you've sold out.

Printing giant HP has used key bloggers to help transmit their latest message – often in the form of a new product launch. When choosing a blogger they first use a range of measuring tools, including Twitlevel and Bloglevel to ensure they choose one that will be effective.

Sarah Fortuna, HP's UK and Ireland consumer marketing manager for inkjet and web solutions, said: 'We need to see that a blog is fresh and that it fits whatever criteria we have chosen. We also ask what benefit we can bring to the blogger.'

So when they have a fresh gadget to tell the world about, getting bloggers to talk freely about it is an important part of their promotional strategy.

Reviews

Reviews are a different beastie altogether. It might not seem that way at first, when you get sent free stuff to try out, but they are. Reviews are when you sample, test or trial something and give your honest opinion of it. Once again, it's nothing new, only a new way of doing it. Mainstream media is awash with books, CDs, DVDs, face creams, foodstuffs and other goodies clamouring to be reviewed. Journalists do not pay for them and neither, generally, do their publications. There are noble exceptions to this such as the *Which?* magazines. The freebie fest extends to holidays and prolonged test-drives in fancy cars.

To a blogger it might seem like you've struck a rich seam in the goldmine of booty when you get sent a shiny new such-and-such to review on your blog. Don't be dazzled, it's you who's doing the manufacturer a favour and, as such, you need to keep your review honest. If you really can't think of anything nice to say in your balanced review then consider saying nowt. Talk to your contact with the company, let them know what you're thinking and give them a chance to see if they can resolve matters.

I find it handy to follow a formula with reviews, just so they all get the same treatment. I use the following headings: preamble which includes expectations, initial impressions, what was good, what was bad, overall view and, finally, an attempt to sum up the product in a very short sentence.

It might seem like a gray area – hobbyist bloggers getting free stuff to review – but if you follow guidelines, I don't think it is. Now some schools of thought say bloggers should be clear about what they've been given but I'm not sure it's essential, newspapers don't, do they? That said, I tend to explain what I've been given – or not – to allow the reader to take that into account. For example, if my socks have been knocked off by something I paid cash money for then they'll be double impressed and, conversely, I won't feel so dismayed and cheated by something that turns out to be merely meh if I didn't pay for it.

On my blog I try to stick to reviewing things I would genuinely use and might, under less fortunate circumstances, pay for. On the one hand it may skew my reviews to the favourable as there's a genuine need for whatever it is, but on the other my house, mind and blog aren't getting cluttered up by things I neither want nor require.

There has been much pontification among bloggers and PR types about how this whole business should be approached. It's fair to say the field is fairly new and expanding by the minute, both in size and credibility. I worked for a PR agency for a while and when I left just four and a half years ago, the notion of using bloggers to get a message 'out there' was still considered a bit left field and geeky.

Bloggers also are finding the attention from PR and marketing people bewildering, irritating and dazzling by turn. So, with the advantage of being on both sides of this particular fence, I'd say to keep the following in mind:

- The PR person has a job to do and that is getting the message across for their client. Do expect them to be aware of the basics of you and your blog, but not the detail.
- Remember what the PR person wants from you and what you want from them, but, within that, play nice.
- Poor pitches from PR people happen, they happen to newspapers too. It is annoying but don't waste your energy being furious. If you must, gently point out the errors, but leave it at that.
- The whole social media world is sparkling new and evolving, we are all learning as we go.
- On the off-chance a PR person is reading this, please remember that while most bloggers are amateurs doing this for fun it doesn't make them a total pushover.

Business blogging

So far we've talked about making a bit of money off the back of a blog that primarily fulfils another need. Shortly I'll get round to discussing blogging about your passion in such a way that it might become your fortune too.

Of course, your blog could be your business, if that's what you set out to do. As with anything commercial that's going to work, you need a USP (no not something for the computer, a Unique Selling Point) or a niche (yup, one of them again). It helps to have a clear vision of who your blog visitors are going to be, what they'll get from your blog and, therefore, what you have to offer an advertiser.

Erica Douglas started her blog *Little Mummy* in 2006. Interested in business and entrepreneurship, she read a wide range of blogs on different topics. She said: 'I watched as others built blogs that were making a lot of money. I learned a lot about making money from blogs during that period.'

It was the beginning of her transformation from mummy blogger to mumpreneur. Now her site generates full-time money on part-time hours.

Once Erica reached the fairly attainable level of 100 visitors a day to her blog, she began to get commercial. She sold advertising, text links and sponsored posts. Then Erica realised that the process had taught her a lot of news skills – marketing, writing and sales among them. She packaged up her skills and started to find ways of selling them via new purpose-built blogs. She wrote ebooks and then she created an e-course. 'I realised my number one professional passion is creating e-courses and I've now co-created two e-courses.

'I think anyone is capable of making money from a blog but you need to choose a good niche, build a loyal audience and know how to market it all.'

Erica co-founded *Ace Inspire* with Carol Smith where they offer a range of online business services including an e-course about blogging for business. She runs *Become A Mumpreneur* for parents who want to find new ways of working and *Become A Mummy Blogger* where she offers an e-course on how to get started and keep going.

Of course if you run a business with an online presence, you know I'm going to say that blogging's a pretty good idea too. Freelance blogger and owner of the *Number 1 Writing Agency*,

Fiona Russell, who is hired to write blog posts for other people's business, said: 'Every business should consider a blog for the above reasons. Blogging is a cheap and customer friendly version of marketing, boosting SEO and improving sales/conversions.

'It offers an opportunity for telling potential customers more about a company, for generating greater levels of trust, transparency and authority, as well as offering a platform for promotions and discounts.'

Her clients are business folk who realise that a blog would help their business, but who for various reasons would rather have an expert do it for them. Fiona is delighted to get her teeth into the meat of someone's business to tease out the juicy bits and turn them into blog posts: 'After years in journalism, blogging for myself or other people is a treat. I enjoy finding and revealing the human face of a business. To blog professionally is a dream job.'

So, assuming you don't want to hire someone to write your blog for you, here are some points to think about for your business blog.

- Be yourself. The chances are your customers have 'bought' more than just the fabric of what you offer, they have signed up to you. Give them more of the person behind the business.
- Don't try to sell anything. It sounds a bit back-to-front, but they're already interested enough in your business to read your blog. Instead, share your expertise, some insider's secrets or rationale behind your professional choices.
- Do inform readers about your business. I know I said don't sell, but do tell them about special offers or new products. That's information rather than persuasion.
- Take a little care over what you post. As this is part of your business, there may well be things customers don't want to know about your personal life.
- Style is important. Spelling, grammar and good presentation are going to be fairly important, whatever your line of work.

Online 'expert' CV

While it's fair to say my blog hasn't generated a colossal amount of revenue from ads and sponsored posts – we're thinking dirty weekend in Blackpool rather than luxury cruise in the Caribbean – it has helped give me a leg up to several work opportunities.

As the commercial world wakes up to the power of the blogging voice and the impact of online on their bottom line, business is starting to need blogs and, therefore, bloggers. The wise ones already know that the value of a blog is the credible voice of its author. So bloggers have been approached with offers of putting their internet writing blogging skills out to work.

If you fancy this – whether you want to work with one of the growing band of agencies or directly with a company – there's no reason why you can't polish up your relevant offering, take it with you and offer your services.

Your blog is your CV. 'No it isn't,' I hear you yell, 'my CV is on those slightly dusty A4 sheets in that drawer'. Well. Yes. A great many blogs don't have anything at all to do with the owner's professional life, or, more importantly, the owner's ambitions for their professional life. But some do.

For as long as my long-suffering friends and family can remember, I've been banging on about wanting to write a book. Yes, you know the joke about journalists meeting at a party. One says: 'So I'm writing a book at the moment.' And the other replies. 'Me neither.' However, as you can see, my blog has helped make this happen. And who knows where that'll take me next.

But, back to the CV. Perhaps your passion is, say, making the most astonishingly beautiful and sumptuous cakes, but you don't have the training, experience or inclination to go to catering college and work up from the bottom of the bakery heap. Maybe a few people ask you to make cakes for them. And a few more. Before you know it, you've packed in your day job, got a proper kitchen become a gateaux-preneur. Or a garden designer, or an artist or whatever.

If a potential employer or client gets wind of the genius you are, just make sure that when they find your blog it reinforces what they know. Use it wisely to showcase what you're about. A clear and simple explanation is a good idea; people rapidly cool off when they have to keep on clicking through to get to the buried treasure. Don't make them work for it.

Kath Horwill, has a blog called *Parklover*, which has led her to a change in career: 'I gave up a my full time teaching job in 2009 in order to spend more time with my daughter before she started school. I wanted to use the time as an opportunity to see if I could do something that I had often wished I'd chosen as a career, namely freelance writing.

'My first step was buying *The Greatest Freelance Writing Tips in the World* by Linda Jones. Linda advised new writers to start a blog so that they had an example of work when pitching editors. I thought that sounded like a great idea, despite the fact that I didn't have much idea about what blogs were.

'I found blogs on various subjects to read and came up with the idea of writing something about my local area, specifically the fantastic parks and playgrounds that I spent vast quantities of time hanging around with my daughter.

'Starting *Parklover* turned out to be a great move. I quickly got involved in the local blogging scene in Manchester and wrote for the *Manchester Literature Festival* blog. Having met the editors of *Creative Tourist*, a Manchester Arts blog, I was commissioned to write a piece on parks for them – my first paid writing work. I now had a number of examples of published work to use in pitches and was able to pitch successfully to write an article for *Running Free* magazine. I've also had fiction published in *Take a Break* magazine and write regularly for the parenting website *Ready for Ten*.

'Writing my blog has brought me all kinds of other opportunities too. I've been able to help publicise various community and charity projects, I've been interviewed on local radio, and met lots of interesting, creative people in the process.'

Resources

Got a question?

Is there a blog life cycle?
Good question. There does seem to be a pattern bloggers follow where they quickly go from first tentative toddles into the blogosphere to becoming infatuated and obsessed, followed by 'burn out' where the energy required to maintain regular enthusiastic posting is more than the energy generated by pleasure and gratification from the process. If you feel fed up with blogging, just stop for a bit – there's no law that says you need to keep going. Have a think about what you're aiming for: will once a week or once a month do? Setting yourself a blog schedule helps some people.

Do I have to run my blog indefinitely?
Of course not. In fact there are some lovely temporary blogs that got abandoned after they served their purpose. A group of deranged friends have just completed a fundraising cycle ride from Land's End to John O'Groats and they blogged to supporters every calloused buttock of the way. Once they got to the top of the country they were happy to put the whole experience behind them, get into a hot bath, and retire the blog. You can read about their adventures as the *Bonking Bikers*.

What do I do about spam?
No, not that nasty pink meaty stuff you used to get at school. Equally unpleasant, but this spam is the boring and unwanted attempts to leave bogus comment on your blog in order to draw traffic to another (commercial) site. Don't allow them space in your brain, just report or delete as appropriate. There are spam filters available, either as part of a blog hosting platform such as Blogger or as a standalone piece of softwear.

Blogging for happiness

What's a spam filter?
It's a way you can choose the level of control you have over comments made on your blog. You can opt to approve all comments before they are made. This means you get to see what someone has said before you allow it to be published. The advantage of this is you only publish what you want while the disadvantage is that readers often want to see their comment instantly and conversation can't flow if they have to wait for you to fiddle around with your computer. You can insist your commenter's key in a code before they are allowed to publish, this, at least, ensures they are real people with eyes and fingers and not computers. I tend to let comments flow freely on new posts, but have a comment approval filter set up for older ones, because that's where the sneaky spammers stick their comments when they think you aren't looking.

How often should I blog?
As often as you like, just don't let it take over your life. I aim to blog three times a week with a bonus photo at the weekend, but, who said I was a good example?

What's RSS?
It stands for really simple syndication. It's the button you can click to get new posts from a blog straight into your feed reader. It's quite important you have one somewhere on your blog so those keen to follow in this manner can do. Make it easy for people to keep track of what you're saying.

What is Flickr?
Flickr is a site that allows you to share your photos. You upload them and decide who can see or use them. Some Flickr users give permission for their photos to be reproduced by others. If you search for images with a creative commons licence you'll find them – just have a look in the advance search section to find details. Generally, if you credit the owner you can use these

pictures but check with each one what the terms are. Other photo-sharing sites are available.

What's Linked Within?
Linked Within is a widget that offers your blog reader a choice of a couple of your previous posts they might like to read once they've finished the fresh one. The idea is to keep readers rooting around in your blog for a bit longer. If someone talks about making a post sticky, that's what they mean – it has stickaround-ability. Other widgets that do similar are available.

What's a blog roll?
Not something you use to wipe your bottom with then? Groan, of course not. It's a list of blogs you like or you think your readers might like that's on the main page of your site. It's very flattering to be included in other people's blogrolls, like being on a Christmas card list but one that everyone knows about.

What's a WOB?
It is white text on a black background, extended to include any light on dark combination. It can look sensational in the hands of a clever designer, but, generally, it's a nightmare to read and gives people headaches. My advice is avoid where possible, even if you think black words on a light background is beyond boring.

What does it mean to trend on Twitter?
Subjects that trend are the ones that are most discussed on Twitter. The top few are listed at the side of the main Twitter page. A quick check of the list will let you know the hot topic of the moment by location. It's a very quick way of keeping abreast of what's exercising the twitterati at any given moment.

What's a hashtag?
It's a short phrase with # in front of it. Tweeters use them to make it easy for other tweeps to follow what's going on. For example, searching a #xfactor hashtag would mean you could

find out what people were saying about the latest must-watch TV without having to wade through other far less important tweets.

What's a tweep?
Someone who tweets, a crowd of them might be refered to as tweeple. It stops feeling really silly after a while.

What is traffic?
It's the number of people who come to your site. If numbers concern you then this number should be as big as possible. The variables include the number of times each person comes and how long they stay for.

What's SEO?
Search Engine Optimisation. It was the very thing you had to know about at the beginning of this latest internet revolution. It means doing everything you can to get your post found by search engine users. Understandably the people who run search engines are somewhat shy about exactly what they use to rank one site above another in a search. And they keep shifting the way they do it to stay ahead of the smarty pants who think they can fiddle the system and get their site to the top of the lists. At first this was something of a dark art and involved putting key phrases into every part of the site so many times the copy became impossible to read comfortably. I wouldn't begin to suggest that SEO is a dying art – there are some very impressive consultants who live well on their skills. However, a common or garden blog shouldn't trouble itself with these matters beyond some basic steps. When you write a heading for a post, make it sum up what the post is about in the simplest terms and give your photos names that relate to the topic rather than 'picture 1'. Use the tags to reiterate what the post is about?

What's a tag?
It's a label you can apply at the end of your post that either reflects the subject or sticks it in a category with other posts. Or both.

Resources

What are links?
This is where readers of your blog can click on a piece of text and get whooshed magically to somewhere else in the internet. Equally, you could be the recipient of an inbound link if someone has referenced and linked to you or one of your posts. They take your readers to something you have mentioned thereby saving them a Google and they are very good for all manner of statistics and ranking witchcraft, especially inbound ones as they show that you're just a little bit popular.

Will I get blogger's block?
It's a common ailment. In extreme cases the blank screen seems to have a life force that prevents any words from being laid down on it. Do not despair, once you crash through the block you'll find your blog mojo has returned with renewed vigour. Here are things you can do to overcome blogger's block:

- Stick a photo up;
- Revisit an old post, especially one of the first ones. I find it helpful to look back to anniversaries, they sometimes inspire;
- See if anyone else is doing something cool and copy it. Don't forget to ask and then credit them with being your inspiration, it's only good manners. Most bloggers are flattered and chuffed to be asked. You might even make a new blogging friend;
- Have some set pieces to return to. I have one or two formats I use in the event of being a bit bleurgh about what to say. You can devise your own. Some of my posts have a 'things I learned' format and others are simply lists... I like lists;
- Interview someone – real or imaginary;
- Do a round-up. Find stuff to share – songs to drive to, TV shows you loved as a child, best things to do while waiting at traffic lights or dishes you know how to cook without looking recipes up, for instance;

Blogging for happiness

- Review something – was there something you experienced recently that is worth telling the world about?
- Just start writing and see what happens. You might be surprised by what comes out. You don't need to publish it, but I'll bet you find something to say.

What's html?
Hyper text marker language is the code that is used to create web pages. However, mercifully, it's not necessary to understand it – just that it exists. I equate it to my car. I can drive it and I have the vaguest notion that it isn't little pixies under the bonnet drinking diesel and pushing the wheels round but after that I'm stumped.

What are all these badges?
You might have noticed that some of the blogs you visit have some logos on them. These badges indicate all the things the blog is involved with – some even show that the blog has been a winner – or contender – in some kind of competition. Some bloggers are clearly so thrilled with them that their blogs positively bristle with them, flashing and twinkling away. Now they are a lovely thing, but in order that your readers aren't rendered catatonic by the hypnotic effects of dozens, I would counsel a little moderation.

Web 2.0, where do I get it?
You can't get it and if you don't know that you obviously haven't got it. Web 2.0 is what's used to describe the current attitude of the internet where sharing and quality content are all important. Think not what can the internet do for me but what can I do for the people of the web. And some form of eKarma will work to bring you what you really want.

Metrics, isn't that a character in a film?
It might be, but I couldn't get very far through the film before I was utterly bewildered and had to give up. Oh, that was *The Matrix!* Metrics are also utterly bewildering to me, but I under-

stand they are the calculations and formulae used to evaluate all sorts of clever internet things. They include things like the number of people who visit your site, where they came from, how long they stay, what they look at, how many sites link to your site and how influential they are. It also takes in connections to Twitter, Facebook and such like.

And algorithms?
These are the almost mystical sequences of calculations and measurements used by the likes of Google to decide who they pick and rank the pages they offer searchers. They are shrouded in secrecy and prone to changes – all you need to know is they exist. Less covertly they are used to determine league tables such as the Tots 100.

Rankings, wasn't that a crime writer?
Not the creator of Rebus the detective, that's Ian Rankin, but lists of blogs or twitters collated according to metrics and algorithms.

What's a vlog?
Vlog is what happens when you mix video with blog. See v-log. It's now so easy to create a film clip on a phone or small camera and it's a piece of proverbial cake to edit it and put it online. Many bloggers – especially those for whom writing isn't enjoyable – prefer to vlog. There are also some show-and-tell type situations where nothing but moving pictures will do.

What's a meme?
It's like a theme on the internet that passes from one blogger to another. In some cases there's a standard form all the posts adopt and in others they invite blogging friends to participate, pick up the baton if you like. It's nothing as intimidating and complicated as the name might suggest.

What are page views?
This is the number of times a particular page is clicked on.

What is a SAHM/WAHM?
Stay at home mother or work at home mother. More shorthand from the text and twitter generation. I also hold Twitter responsible for ensuring the permanence of LOL (laugh out loud), LMAO (laughing my arse off), ROFL (rolling on the floor laughing), OH (other half), DH (darling husband), DS (darling son), DD (darling daughter). I've often wondered at those talented folk who can tweet while they roll on the floor, I certainly couldn't.

When is a book an e-book?
When it is published electronically and available, therefore, to read online, on a computer or on a reader such as Kindle.

Why do bloggers' children have such peculiar names?
Do you mean mine Boy One, Boy Two and Boy Three? I thought it was easier in the long run... No? It's to protect the kids' privacy and identity. Lots of bloggers do it using initials or pet names instead of the real one. Although now I come to think of it...

Where do I learn how to do the blog hop?
It's not like salsa, there aren't classes. Actually it's simple – it's when you read and comment on one blog before moving on to the next. It is one of various ways of socialising your blog with those of others. In the case of a link you can use something like a Linky Tool to help – it provides a list on the bottom of a post where bloggers can add their contribution. Alternatively you can simply ask participants to supply links to their blogs in your comments boxes.

And what about the blogging carnival?
Before you rush to put on your elaborate feathered head dress (unless you really want to) it's a name given to a blog post that references, and links to, many other posts by other bloggers. In some circles it may be known as a roundup and may have a

specific, possibly topical, theme. A carnival will be announced, for example I might say I'm going to hold one for, oh, all the funny thing that have resulted from falling over in public. I'll pass the message on through blogs, forums, Twitter and Facebook and a rash of hilarious posts will flood in. I'll incorporate links to them into a trippy stumbly post that rounds them all up.

Should reveal my blog stats?
Well, would you reveal your other statistics? Somehow disclosing blog stats – that is the number of people who visit your site – has taken on the same taboo as blabbing about your salary or what the scales tell you in the morning. That said, in most cases, it's hardly life and death so, I'd say, it's up to you.

What's a GIF?
It stands for Graphics Interchange Format and is those constantly moving images you find all over the web. Occasionally cute or effective but mostly annoying.

What is a semantic link?
It's when you use a section of text as the click-on bit for a link to another page, the text tells the clicker about the site they are being taken to. It helps search engine magic no end and is much better than saying 'click HERE for more information'.

URL?
This is the uniform resource locator of a web page. Every time you make a new blog post you create a URL – it's basically the address on the internet of the page you have generated.

What happens when something goes viral?
Something – a post, photo or video – has suddenly become popular online and is being passed from person via various social media means. It includes videos, blog posts or news items.

Wifi?
It's a standard way of connecting wirelessly to the internet.

Blogging for happiness

And aggregation?
It is a website or piece of software that collects similar information from various sources and delivers it.

Bloggers recommend / quoted
I would like to thank the fabulous bloggers who helped me write this book. Their ideas, suggestions and inspiration kept me going.

Heather B. Armstrong – *Dooce.com*
Aspie In The Family – *aspieinthefamily.com*
Sheila Averbuch – *stopwatchgardener.com*
Cas Baillie – *frugalfamily.co.uk*
Jorn Barger – *Robotwisdom.com*
Paula Battle – *battlingon.wordpress.com*
Alan Baxter – *alanbaxteronline.com* (*The Word*)
Belle de Jour – *belledejour-uk.blogspot.com*
Rebecca Blood – *rebeccablood.net* (*Rebecca's Pocket*)
Jax Blunt – *liveotherwise.co.uk/makingitup* (*Making It Up*)
Bonking Bikers – *thebonkingbikers.wordpress.com*
Kathryn Brown – *crystaljigsaw.blogspot.com*
Bumbling – *bumblingalong.wordpress.com*
Trish Burgess – *mumsgoneto.blogspot.com*
Sandy Calico – *sandycalico.blogspot.com* (*Baby Baby*)
Alice Castle – *dulwichdivorcee.com*
Caz – *cazandbelle.blogspot.com* (*After Anabelle*)
Tamsin Constable – *mumblog.net* (*Looking For Dragons*)
Jayne Crammond – *jaynelc.wordpress.com* (*Mum's The Word*)
Gordon Darroch – *gordondarroch.wordpress.com* (*Unreal Domain*)
Gordon Darroch – *autisticdad.blogspot.com*
Gordon Darroch – *wordsforpress.wordpress.com*
Adrian Doherty – *adriandoherty.blogspot.com* (*Earthy Android*)
Erica Douglas – *Littlemummy.com*
Josie George – *sleepisfortheweak.org.uk*
Nadine Hill – *Jugglemum.com* (*Time Management Mum*)

Kath Horwill – *parklover.wordpress.com*
Jennifer Howze – *jenography.net*
Liz Jarvis – *themumblog.com*
Jay – *Mochabeaniemummy.com*
Thea Jolly – *theajolly.wordpress.com* (*A Talent For Living*)
Kate – *gigglingatitall.blogspot.com*
Keith Kendrick – *reluctanthousedad.com*
Eva Keogan – *Nixdminx.com*
Caron Lindsay – *carons-musings.blogspot.com*
Hamish McFarlane – *difficultsecondnovel.com*
Sheonad Macfarlane – *touchandtickle.blogspot.com*
Peter Merholz – *peterme.com*
Christine Mosler – *christinemosler.wordpress.com* (*Thinly Spread*)
Nickie O'Hara – *iamtypecast.com*
Victoria Pires – *glowstars.net*
Dr Rant – *drrant.net*
Mike Ritchie – *mikeritchiemedia-comesatime.blogspot.com*
Nomita – *ebabee*
Allison Rosser – *cancerandbabyequalschaos.blogspot.com*
Fiona Russell – *fionaoutdoors.com*
Fiona Russell – *thenumberonewritingagency.co.uk*
Susanne Scott – *amodernmother.com*
Rosie Scribble – *rosiescribble.typepad.com*
Sara – *Walkingwithangels.co.uk*
Sian To – *mummy-tips.com*
Carol Smith – *dancewithoutsleep.co.uk*
Susanne – *ghostwritermummy.wordpress.com*
Tilly – *tillytatas.blogspot.com*
Tracy T – *beadspaperglue.blogspot.com*
Dil Uppal – *scform.com* (*Skincare For Men*)
Ryan Wenstrup-Moore – *transatlanticblonde.blogspot.com*
Sally Whittle – *whosthemummy.co.uk*
Maggy Woodley – *redtedart.com*

Blogging for happiness

Bibliography
I Know Why The Caged Bird Sings, Maya Angelou
The Weblog Handbook, Rebecca Blood
Women's Room, Marilyn French
Pollyanna, Eleanor H. Porter
Threeplay, Hamish McFarlane
Harry Potter and the Philosophers Stone, J.K. Rowling
The Colour of Magic, Sir Terry Pratchett
Desiderata of Happiness, Max Ehrmann
I Don't Have Time To Write, Nadine Hill
The Greatest Freelance Writing Tips in the World, Linda Jones

Useful websites
Aceinspire.com – Erica Douglas and Antonia Chitty offer courses in using the internet for business
Affiliate window.com – brings bloggers and brands together
birthtraumaassociation.org.uk – charity for people traumatised by childbirth
Blogger.com – free place to set up a blog
Blogher.com – giant American network for female bloggers
blogscanada.ca – Canadian blogging network
blogs.com.au – Australian blogging network
britmums.com – network for British blogging mums and dads
clickbank.com – a business linking brands and bloggers
dalerockell.com – confidence and achievement coach
ebuzzing.co.uk – linking brands and social media
e-junkie.com – helping you sell online
glammedia.com – marketing through social media
handpickedmedia.com – social media agency and collective of independent blogs
hotter.com – comfy shoes
kiwiology.co.nz – New Zealand blog network
maternitymatters.net – blog about birth trauma
mentalhealth.org.uk – mental health charity in UK

Resources

mind.org.uk – mental health charity in UK
mooddisorderscanada.ca – mental health charity in Canada
oft.gov.uk – Office of Fair Trade, UK Government department
picnik.com – free photo manipulation software
pingomatic.com – service that tells search engines there's a new post
readyforten.com – a site for parents of primary aged children
savethechildren.org.uk – children's charity in the UK
scottishroundup.co.uk – weekly selection of Scottish blogs
stv.tv – website of Scotland's main broadcaster
terribodell.com – clinical psychotherapist
topblogs.ca – Canadian blog network
tots100.co.uk – site that ranks top British parenting bloggers
unicef.org.uk – leading children's charity
webbyawards.com – internet awards
wordpress.com – blogging platform

Index

Ace Inspire 123
Adaptive Path 5
AdSense 116
Affiliate Futures 119
Affiliate Window 119, 138
aggregation 136
algorithms 78, 133
Allan, (Lord) R. 6
Amazon 119
Angelou, M. (*I Know Why The Caged Bird Sings*) 17
Armstrong, H. B. (*Dooce*) 94
Asperger's Syndrome 34, 46, 65, 66
Aspie in the Family 66
autism 34, 64–5, 66
Averbuch, S. (*Stopwatch Gardener*) 36, 43

Baillie, C. (*Frugalfamily*) 68–9
balance 21, 22, 99, 102
Barger, J. 5–6
Battle, P. (*Battling On*) 87
Baxter, A. (*Realmshift, Magesign* and *The Word*) 13–14
Become A Mummy Blogger 123
Become A Mumpreneur 123
Belle de Jour 90
bereavement 38; *see also* loss (of a loved one); grief; miscarriage
birth trauma 24–5, 138; *see also* trauma
blip 72
blog categories 15, 68, 78, 83
blog community *see* community (online)
Blogger.com 6, 59, 74
Bloggers for Vision 48
blog hop 134

Blogonymous 87–8
blog roll 75–6, 79, 129
Blood, R. (*Weblog Handbook* and *Rebecca's Pocket*) 6, 7–8
Blunt, J. (*Making It Up*) 28
Bodell, T. 8, 20–1, 22, 32, 33, 35, 38, 98, 102
Britmums 10, 30–1, 35, 55, 83
Brown, K. (*Crystal Jigsaw*) 14–15
Brown, S. 103
Bumbling 39, 87, 88–9, 90, 99
Burgess, T. (*Mum's Gone To...*) 63

Calico, S. (*Baby Baby* and *Parent Confidential*) 12, 87
carnival 55, 134–5
Castle, A. (*Dulwich Divorcee*) 12–13
categories (of blog) 15, 68, 78, 83
Caz (*After Anabelle*) 67
children 96, 134
Clayton, H. 118
Click Bank 119
comments 10, 35, 62, 69, 93
community (online) 10, 12, 24–5, 28–40, 43, 52, 65, 75, 82, 88, 91, 102, 115; see also international blog communities
confidence, lack of 53, 105
confidentiality 94, 100
confrontation 98
Constable, T. (*Looking for Dragons*) 29, 68
conversation 35
copyright 75, 76, 92
creativity 8, 11, 40–2, 126
Cybermummy 31, 91, 103
Cyhlarova. E. 34, 48

Darroch, G. (*Unreal Domain*, *Autistic Dad* and *Words For Press*) 62, 106
Del.icio.us 72

Index

depression 1, 3, 20, 22, 32, 40, 50, 86, 88, 95; *see also* mental health
diary 4–5, 7–8, 23, 56, 63, 67, 93
Digg 72
Doherty, A. (*Earthy Android*) 70
Douglas, E. (*Littlemummy*) 115, 123
Dr. Rant 26–7

e-book 134
eBuzz 114, 118
Ehrmann, M. (*Desederata of Happiness*) 105
eJunkie 119
Emily (*Mummy Limited*) 87

Facebook 6, 57, 70, 72, 93, 103, 107
feminism 8
Feminist Fridays 8
Flickr 75, 128
Fortuna, S. 120
French, M. (*Women's Room*) 9

Gallson, D. 38–9
George, J. (*Sleep is for the Weak*) 50
GIF 135
Glam Media 113, 115, 118, 138
Google Analytics 77
Google+ 70, 72
grief 1, 38, 66–7; *see also* bereavement; loss

Handpicked Community 115
Handpicked Media 115, 118, 138
headlines 73
Hill, N. (*I Don't Have Time To Write*) 111
Horwill, K. (*Parklover*) 126
Hotter Shoes 119
Howze, J. (*Jenography* and *Alpha Mummy*) 31, 66

Blogging for Happiness

HP 120
html 132
Hughes, D. (*All That Comes With It*) 51–2

international blog communities 30
isolation 12, 29, 32, 36

Jarvis, L. (*The Mum Blog*) 83–4
Jay (*Mocha Beanie Mummy*) 87
Jayne (*Mum's The Word*) 25
Jolly, T. (*Talent For Living*) 19
Jones, L. (*The Greatest Freelance Writing Tips In The World*) 126
Joseph Salmon Trust 51
journalism 41, 117, 121

Kate (*Giggling At It All*) 40
keepsake 68–9
Kendrick, K. (*Chronicles Of A Reluctant Housedad*) 18–19, 101–2
Keogan, E. (*Nixdminx*) 50
klout 71, 78

Lindsay, C. (*Caron's Musings*) 15, 22
Linked-In 72
Linked Within 129
links 75, 131, 135
Linky 71
loss (of a loved one) 1, 2, 19, 38, 66–7, 86; *see also* bereavement; grief; miscarriage

Madden, K. (*Beautyandthedirt.com*) 115
McFarlane, H. (*Threeplay* and *Difficult Second Novel*) 42
Macfarlane, S. (*Touch And Tickle*) 22–3
Magnanti, Dr. B. 90
Maternity Matters 25
meme 71, 133
mental health 1, 5, 34, 40, 62, 86, 96; *see also* depression

Index

Mental Health Foundation 34, 48
mental illness 1
Merholz, P. 5–6
metrics 132
Mind 23
miscarriage 2, 36 50, 64, 71, 95; *see also* loss (of a loved one); bereavement; grief
Mocha Beanie Mummy 56
Mood Disorders Society of Canada 38
Mosler, C. (*Thinly Spread*) 50
mummy blog 60, 98

networks 70
niche 62, 65, 114, 123
Nickie (*Typecast*) 87
Nomita (*Ebabee*) 64
Number 1 Writing Agency 123

Office of Fair Trading (OFT) 118
online diary 4–5, 7–8, 23, 56, 63, 67, 93

page views 133
Peer-Index 78
pictures 74, 76, 96
Pires, V. (*Glowstars*) 48
planning 111
Pollyanna 17
positive thinking 19, 20
PR 122
privacy 91

rankings 78, 133
Ready for Ten 46, 126
Reddit 72
Ritchie, M. (*There Comes A Time*) 28
Rockell, D. 11, 33, 40

Rosie Scribbles 50
Rosser, A. (*Cancer And Baby Equals Chaos*) 67
RSS 74, 128
Russell, F. (*Fionaoutdoors*) 46

safety 98
Sara (*Walking With Angels*) 66
Save the Children 50
ScottishRoundup 30
Scott, S. (*A Modern Mother*) 31, 84
self hosting 61
self knowledge 47
semantic link 135
SEO 71, 124, 130
short term blogs 127
Silent Sunday 56
Smith, C. (*Parent Panel*, *New Mummy's Tips* and *Dance Without Sleeping*) 113
spam 127–8
stigma 39
StumbleUpon 70
STV 82–3
Susanne (*Ghostwritermummy*) 24, 25

tag 130
Technorati 77, 78
Tilly (*Tilly Tatas*) 64
To, S. (*Mummy-Tips*) 31, 50
Tots100 78
Tracy T. (*Beadspaperglue*) 31
traffic 13, 48, 62, 74, 78, 79, 80, 81, 82, 114, 127, 130
trauma 67; *see also* birth trauma
truth 99
Tweeps 109, 130
Twitter 54, 57, 70, 72, 76
    follow 108

Index

   #FF 108
   hashtag 108, 129
   retweet (RT) 108
   trend 129
typepad 74

UNICEF 50
updating 74
Uppal, D. (*Skincare For Men*) 41
URL 135

viral 135
Vision's Gold Challenge 48
vlog 4, 111, 133

Web 2.0 132
Webbies 83
Web log 5
Wenstrup-Moore, R. (*Transatlantic Blonde*) 8
whistleblowing 27
Whittle, S. (*Who's The Mummy?*) 79
wifi 135
Wikio 78
WOB 129
Woodley, M. (*Red Ted Art*) 80
Wordpress 59, 74
worries 23
writing, benefits of 8, 23

Lightning Source UK Ltd.
Milton Keynes UK
UKOW041808301212

204232UK00001B/2/P